MW01106273

DxRx:
Heart Failure

Theo E. Meyer, MBChB, FCP(SA), DPhil

Director, Advanced Heart Failure Program
Professor of Medicine
University of Massachusetts Medical School
Worcester, MA

Dennis A. Tighe, MD, FACC, FACP

University of Massachusetts Medical Center
Associate Professor of Medicine
Associate Director, Noninvasive Cardiology
University of Massachusetts Medical School
Worcester, MA

Series Editor: Dennis A. Tighe, MD, FACC, FACP

JONES AND BARTLETT PUBLISHERS
Sudbury, Massachusetts
BOSTON   TORONTO   LONDON   SINGAPORE

World Headquarters
Jones and Bartlett Publishers
40 Tall Pine Drive
Sudbury, MA 01776
978-443-5000
info@jbpub.com
www.jbpub.com

Jones and Bartlett Publishers Canada
2406 Nikanna Road
Mississauga, ON L5C 2W6
Canada

Jones and Bartlett Publishers International
Barb House, Barb Mews
London W6 7PA
United Kingdom

Production Credits
Executive Publisher: Christopher Davis
Production Manager: Amy Rose
Associate Production Editor: Carolyn F. Rogers
Editorial Assistant: Kathy Richardson
Marketing Manager: Matthew Payne
Cover Design: Anne Spencer
Composition: ATLIS
Printing and Binding: Malloy, Inc.
Cover Printing: Malloy, Inc.

Library of Congress Cataloging-in-Publication Data
Meyer, Theo E.
 Dx/Rx : heart failure / Theo E. Meyer, Dennis A. Tighe.
  p. ; cm.
 ISBN 0-7637-2309-6 (pbk. : alk. paper)
 1. Heart failure—Handbooks, manuals, etc.
 [DNLM: 1. Heart Failure, Congestive—Handbooks. WG 39 M613d 2005]
I. Title: Heart failure. II. Tighe, Dennis A. III. Title.
 RC685.C53M49 2005
 616.1′29—dc22

                                                        2004022749

The authors, editor, and publisher have made every effort to provide accurate information. However, they are not responsible for errors, omissions, or for any outcomes
related to the use of the contents of this book and take no responsibility for the use
of the products described. Treatments and side effects described in this book may
not be applicable to all patients; likewise, some patients may require a dose or experience a side effect that is not described herein. The reader should confer with his or
her own physician regarding specific treatments and side effects. Drugs and medical
devices are discussed that may have limited availability controlled by the Food and
Drug Administration (FDA) for use only in a research study or clinical trial. The drug
information presented has been derived from reference sources, recently published
data, and pharmaceutical research data. Research, clinical practice, and government
regulations often change the accepted standard in this field. When consideration is
being given to use of any drug in the clinical setting, the healthcare provider or
reader is responsible for determining FDA status of the drug, reading the package
insert, reviewing prescribing information for the most up-to-date recommendations
on dose, precautions, and contraindications, and determining the appropriate usage
for the product. This is especially important in the case of drugs that are new or
seldom used.

Printed in the United States of America
08 07 06 05 04   10 9 8 7 6 5 4 3 2 1

Table of Contents

Editor's Preface

Heart failure is a syndrome caused by a variety of processes. A substantial number of Americans currently live with heart failure and, as our population continues to age and patients with underlying cardiac diseases experience increasing longevity, the medical community will be faced with a growing epidemic of heart failure. In this monograph, Dr. Meyer and I describe the epidemiology and etiologies of heart failure along with the important aspects of diagnosis and management of patients with this syndrome. The text presents this information in a succinct and direct manner and is supplemented by very informative tables and figures. I am most grateful to Dr. Meyer for sharing his vast experience and valuable insights into the care of patients with heart failure and for an excellent contribution to this series.

Dennis A. Tighe
Worcester, MA

Preface

Heart failure is a clinical syndrome that is usually characterized by signs or symptoms of intravascular or interstitial fluid excess, including shortness of breath, rales, and edema; fatigue and decreased exercise tolerance; or the combination of these manifestations. The clinical syndrome of heart failure is caused by a wide variety of disorders that includes valvular, myocardial, pericardial, and other noncardiac diseases. Thirty to fifty percent of patients presenting with signs and symptoms of heart failure have a normal left ventricular ejection fraction; the term for this clinical state is diastolic HF. Over the last decade, there have been significant developments toward the early recognition of preclinical heart failure states, the modification of the natural history of left ventricular dysfunction by using neurohumoral blockade, and the implementation of disease management programs to effectively manage this chronic disabling syndrome.

The purpose of this manual is to present a pragmatic, user-friendly review of all aspects of the diagnosis and management of heart failure. The text is tightly organized into a bulleted outline to avoid redundancy. The text is further supplemented by appropriate tables, figures, and salient references, which are intended to summarize important clinical data and current professional society recommendations and provide the reader with additional reading material.

I wish to thank my coauthor, Dennis A. Tighe, for his help and excellent contribution to this manual.

Theo E. Meyer
Worcester, MA

CHAPTER 1

Introduction

■ Definition and Classification of Heart Failure

- Heart failure (HF) is a clinical syndrome that is usually characterized by signs or symptoms of intravascular or interstitial fluid excess, including shortness of breath, rales, and edema; fatigue and decreased exercise tolerance; or the combination of these manifestations.

- The term *HF* is preferred over the commonly used *congestive HF* because many patients with HF may only complain of decreased exercise tolerance rather than congestive symptoms.

- The clinical syndrome of HF is caused by a wide variety of disorders, which include valvular, myocardial, pericardial, and other noncardiac diseases.[1]

- Thirty to fifty percent of patients presenting with signs and symptoms of HF have a normal left ventricular ejection fraction (LVEF); the term for this clinical state is *diastolic HF.*

- Acute HF with pulmonary edema is one of the most common and devastating consequences of acute left ventricular (LV) dysfunction. Increased pulmonary venous pressure accompanying LV failure causes transudation of fluid into the pulmonary capillary interstitium, which limits the transfer of oxygen from alveoli into blood.

  • The resulting hypoxia, and sometimes acidosis, can lead to a further decrease in body tissue oxygenation. Pulmonary edema is likely to be the most frequent cause of acute respiratory failure in critically ill patients.

- Terms used to describe the various HF syndromes are defined in Table 1-1.

Table 1-1: Definitions of Preclinical and Clinical Heart Failure Syndromes

Preclinical systolic dysfunction:
   Asymptomatic patients who have impaired systolic LV dysfunction with an ejection fraction of less than 40%

Preclinical diastolic dysfunction:
   Asymptomatic patients with a normal ejection fraction who have impaired diastolic LV dysfunction as assessed by cardiac catheterization or by Doppler echocardiography

Systolic heart failure:
   Symptomatic patients who have impaired systolic dysfunction (an ejection fraction of less than 40%)

Diastolic heart failure:
   Symptomatic patients with heart failure and an ejection fraction of greater than 40%

Acute heart failure:
   Clinical syndrome characterized by a sudden onset of reduced organ perfusion in association with pulmonary congestion

Chronic heart failure:
   Clinical syndrome in which abnormal systolic or diastolic LV function is associated with a constellation of secondary changes in other organs, leading to congestion or exercise limitation or both

■ Prevalence and Incidence of HF

- Almost 5 million Americans have HF. Increasing prevalence and increasing hospitalizations and deaths resulting from HF have made HF a major chronic health care issue in the United States and other developed countries.[2–6]
- The magnitude of the problem of HF is large now, and it is expected to become much larger.
  - As more and more cardiac patients are able to survive and live longer with their diseases, their opportunities for developing HF increase.
  - Future growth in the elderly population will likely result in increasing numbers of persons with this condition regardless of trends in coronary disease morbidity and mortality.

- HF is the most common diagnosis in hospital patients aged 65 years and older. HF is present in almost 1.4 million persons under 60 years of age. HF is present in 2% of persons aged 40 to 59, more than 5% of persons aged 60 to 69, and 10% of persons aged 70 and older.
- Prevalence is at least 25% greater among the black population than among the white population.
- HF is twice as common in persons with hypertension compared with normotensive persons, and it is five times more common in persons who have had a myocardial infarction compared to persons who have not.[2]
  - Normal LVEF is often found in persons with HF and is more common in women than in men.[7]
- Over the past 50 years, the incidence of HF has declined among women, but not among men.[8]

Risk Factors for the Development of HF

- *Hypertension* is the most common risk factor for HF. It confers twice the risk of HF and also carries the highest population-attributable risk among all risk factors for HF.
  - Systolic, diastolic blood pressure and pulse pressure are related to the risk of HF, but the relation is strongest for systolic and pulse pressure.[9]
- *Diabetics* have about a twofold to eightfold greater risk of HF than those without diabetes.
- Patients with *coronary artery disease* and asymptomatic patients with *impaired LV systolic function* have a fourfold to fivefold greater risk of HF than patients without coronary disease and patients with normal LV function.
- Other risk factors leading to HF include the use of certain chemotherapeutic agents for the treatment of cancers, alcohol abuse, chronic valvular disease, and uncontrolled tachycardia.

Prognosis of HF

- Survival following the diagnosis of congestive HF is less likely in men than women, yet, even in women, only about 20% survive much longer than 8 to 12 years. The outlook is not much better than that for most forms of cancer. The fatality rate of HF is high, with one in five persons dying within 1 year.[10]

- The median survival time for patients with HF is 1.7 years for men and 3.2 years for women. After 5 years, only 25% of men and 38% of women surveyed remained alive, and these figures fell to 11% and 21%, respectively, after 10 years.

- Although HF patients with normal LVEF have a lower mortality risk than patients with reduced LVEF, they have four times the mortality risk of control subjects who are free of HF.[11]

- Sudden death is common in these patients and occurs at a rate of six to nine times that of the general population.

- Recent data have shown that survival rates for male and female patients with HF have improved.

■ Etiology of HF

- Coronary artery disease is the underlying cause of HF in approximately two thirds of patients with LV systolic dysfunction. The remaining, nonischemic causes of HF may be identifiable (e.g., hypertension, valvular disease, myocardial toxins, or myocarditis) or unidentifiable (e.g., idiopathic dilated cardiomyopathy).

- Seventy percent of men and 78% of women with HF had an antecedent diagnosis of hypertension, while 40% of both men and women had a prior history of both hypertension and coronary disease. Prevalent coronary disease was less common in women than in men.

- Approximately 75% of patients requiring admission to a hospital for acute LV failure, other than those patients who developed HF from an evolving myocardial infarction, are likely to have received treatment for HF in the past, and almost half of these patients will have experienced chest pain with the acute episode.

- Lists of the etiologies of HF are shown in Tables 1-2 and 1-3.

Table 1-2:   Etiology of Heart Failure

Etiology	Percentage of patients (%)
Coronary artery disease	51
Nonischemic causes	49
Etiology uncertain (idiopathic)	32
Etiology established	17
Valvular	4
Hypertension	4
Ethanol	2
Viral	<1
Postpartum	<1
Amyloidosis	<1
Other (chemotherapeutic agents)	8

Table 1-3:   Causes of Acute Heart Failure and Pulmonary Edema

Myocardial disease
- Coronary artery disease
  - Acute myocardial infarction
  - Severe myocardial ischemia
  - Mechanical complications of myocardial infarction
  - Infarction or ischemia on preexisting LV dysfunction
- Hypertrophic heart disease
  - Hypertrophic cardiomyopathy
  - Hypertrophic heart disease of the elderly
- Cardiomyopathy
  - Idiopathic dilated cardiomyopathy
  - Myocarditis
  - Post bypass LV pump dysfunction

Valvular heart disease
- Aortic regurgitation
- Mitral regurgitation
- Mitral stenosis
- Atrial myxoma
- Aortic stenosis

Hypertensive heart disease
- Hypertensive crisis

■ Hospitalization Rates

- The number of hospital discharges of patients with HF today is almost five times greater than it was twenty-five years ago.
- Repeat hospitalizations for patients with HF are a relatively frequent occurrence within a short period of time following hospital discharge. The six-month readmission rate varies from 36% to 50%.[12,13]

■ Economic Costs

- In the United States, the total direct economic costs devoted to the management of HF is estimated to exceed $30 billion, based on hospitalizations for this condition, physicians' office visits, nursing home costs, and treatment modalities annually.[14,15]
  - The economic burden of HF has been calculated to consume approximately 1% of the national health care budgets of countries in Europe.
  - About 75% of the cost is attributable to the high rate of readmissions and the long hospital stays of patients with HF. It is estimated that about half of the cost can be saved through prudent outpatient management of HF.

■ References

1. Gaasch WH, Blaustein AS, LeWinter MM. Heart Failure and clinical disorders of left ventricular diastolic function. In: Gaasch WH, LeWinter MM, eds. *Left Ventricular Diastolic Dysfunction and Heart Failure.* Philadelphia, PA: Lea & Febiger; 1994:245-258.

2. Schocken DD, Arrieta MI, Leaverton PE, Ross EA. Prevalence and mortality rate of congestive heart failure in the United States. *J Am Coll Cardiol.* 1992;20:301-306.

3. Rodeheffer RJ, Jacobsen SJ, Gersh BJ, et al. The incidence and prevalence of congestive heart failure in Rochester, Minnesota. *Mayo Clin Proc.* 1993;68:1143-1150.

4. National Heart, Lung, and Blood Institute. *Morbidity and mortality chartbook on cardiovascular, lung, and blood diseases.* Bethesda, MD. National Institutes of Health. US Department of Health and Human Services; 1990 and 1994.

5.   Ho KK, Pinsky JL, Kannel WB, Levy D. The epidemiology of heart failure: the Framingham study. *J Am Coll Cardiol.* 1993;22(4 suppl A):6A-13A.

6.   National Center for Health Statistics. National hospital discharge survey. *Vital Health Stat 13.* 1990;12:1-17.

7.   MacCarthy PA, Kearney MT, Nolan J, et al. Prognosis in heart failure with preserved left ventricular systolic function: prospective cohort study. *BMJ.* 2003;327:78-79.

8.   Levy D, Kenchaiah S, Larson MG, et al. Long-term trends in the incidence of and survival with heart failure. *N Engl J Med.* 2002;347:1397-1402.

9.   Haider AW, Larson MG, Franklin SS, Levy D. Framingham Heart Study: systolic blood pressure, diastolic blood pressure, and pulse pressure as predictors of risk for congestive heart failure in the Framingham Heart Study. *Ann Intern Med.* January 7, 2003;138(1):10-16.

10. MacIntyre K, Capewell S, Stewart S, et al. Evidence of improving prognosis in heart failure: trends in case fatality in 66,547 patients hospitalized between 1986 and 1995. *Circulation.* 2000;102:1126-1131.

11. Gustafsson F, Torp-Pedersen C, Brendorp B, Seibaek M, Burchardt H, Kober L. Long-term survival in patients hospitalized with congestive heart failure: relation to preserved and reduced left ventricular systolic function. *Eur Heart J.* 2003;24:863-870.

12. McMurray J, McDonagh T, Morrison CE, Dargie HJ. Trends in hospitalization for heart failure in Scotland, 1980–1990. *Eur Heart J.* 1993;14:1158-1162.

13. Krumholz HM, Parent EM, Tu N, et al. Readmission after hospitalization for congestive heart failure among medicare beneficiaries. *Arch Intern Med.* 1997;157:99-104.

14. O'Connell JB, Bristow MR. Economic impact of heart failure in the United States: a time for a different approach. *J Heart Lung Transplant.* 1994;154:1143-1149.

15. Eriksson H. Heart failure: a growing health care problem. *J Intern Med.* 1995;237:135-141.

CHAPTER 2

Pathophysiology of HF

■ Introduction

- HF is the final common pathway for a number of cardio-vascular conditions that lead to asymptomatic and symptomatic LV systolic and diastolic dysfunction.
- Four stages of HF have been identified by the American Heart Association (details are outlined in Table 2-1)[1]:
  - *Stage A* refers to a patient who is at high risk of developing HF but has no structural disorder of the heart.
  - *Stage B* refers to a patient with a structural disorder of the heart but who has not yet developed symptoms of HF.
  - *Stage C* refers to a patient with past or current symptoms of HF associated with underlying structural heart disease.
  - *Stage D* refers to a patient with end-stage disease who requires specialized treatment strategies, such as mechanical circulatory support, continuous inotropic infusions, cardiac transplantation, or hospice care.
- The syndrome of HF is the consequence of a number of primary and secondary changes in response to an inciting process, such as chamber dilation and structural remodeling of the LV chamber, impaired myocyte shortening, neurohumoral activation, systemic vasoconstriction, and sodium retention.
- HF is associated with a spectrum of varying degrees of systolic and diastolic LV dysfunction (Figure 2-1).

■ Chamber Remodeling

- Cardiac chambers alter their size and geometry in response to chronic changes in hemodynamic load. Long-standing pressure overload (as a consequence of

Table 2-1: Stages of Heart Failure

Stage	Description	Examples
A	Patients at high risk of developing HF because of the presence of conditions that are strongly associated with the development of HF (Such patients have no identified structural or functional abnormalities of the pericardium, myocardium, or cardiac valves and have never shown signs or symptoms of HF.)	Systemic hypertension; coronary artery disease; diabetes mellitus; history of cardiotoxic drug therapy or alcohol abuse; personal history of rheumatic fever; family history of cardiomyopathy
B	Patients who have developed structural heart disease that is strongly associated with the development of HF but who have never shown signs or symptoms of HF	LV hypertrophy or fibrosis; LV dilatation or hypocontractility; asymptomatic valvular heart disease; previous myocardial infarction
C	Patients who have current or prior symptoms of HF associated with underlying structural heart disease	Dyspnea or fatigue caused by LV systolic dysfunction; asymptomatic patients who are undergoing treatment for prior symptoms of HF
D	Patients with advanced structural heart disease and marked symptoms of HF at rest despite maximal medical therapy and who require specialized interventions	Patients who are frequently hospitalized for HF or cannot be safely discharged from the hospital; patients in the hospital awaiting heart transplantation; patients at home receiving continuous intravenous support for symptom relief or being supported with a mechanical circulatory assist device; patients in a hospice setting for the management of HF

HF indicates heart failure

From: Hunt SA, Baker DW, Chin MH, et al. ACC/AHA guidelines for the evaluation and management of chronic heart failure in the adult: executive summary. *Circulation.* 2001;104:2996-3007.

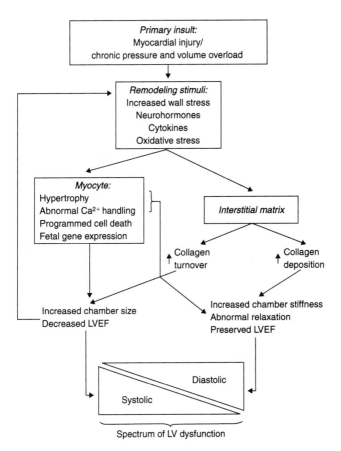

Figure 2.1: Depicted is the sequence of events and factors that mediate the transition from the primary cardiac insult to LV dysfunction. Remodeling stimuli alter myocyte size, physiology, and genes, as well as the interstitial matrix. This leads to a decrease in systolic chamber function and abnormalities in diastolic function.

either aortic stenosis or hypertension) or prolonged volume overload (for example, as a result of chronic mitral regurgitation) leads to remodeling of the LV chamber. The chamber remodels in direct relation to the imposed hemodynamic burden (Figure 2-1).

- A specific type of remodeling occurs as a result of myocardial infarction (Figure 2-2).[2]

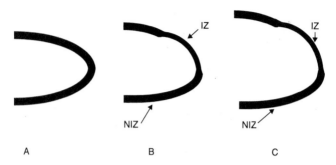

Figure 2.2: The schematic representation shows the changes in LV geometry (remodeling), from the normal shaped heart (A) to 24 hours (B) and 6 weeks (C) after myocardial infarction. Note the changes in the infarct zone (IZ) and noninfarct zone (NIZ) over time.

- Remodeling in response to pathological conditions can initially be considered to be adaptive, but, over a period of time, these changes become maladaptive and eventually progress to chamber and myocardial dysfunction, usually associated with significant ventricular enlargement.
- Right and left ventricular dilation often leads to more than mild mitral and tricuspid regurgitation.

◼ Neurohumoral Activation

- Structural abnormalities of the heart are of paramount importance in generating the clinical disorder. However, the changes in extracardiac neurohumoral systems contribute to the progression of HF and the exercise limitation associated with HF.[3]
- Neurohumoral responses include activation of the sympathetic nervous and the renin-angiotensin systems and increased release of antidiuretic hormone (vasopressin) and atrial natriuretic peptide.[3–7] The net effect of these neurohumoral responses is the onset of arterial vasoconstriction (to help maintain blood pressure), venous constriction (increased venous pressure), and increased blood volume.

- In general, these neurohumoral responses can be viewed as compensatory mechanisms, but they can also aggravate HF by promoting programmed myocyte death, myonecrosis, myocyte hypertrophy, interstitial myocardial fibrosis, and chamber dilatation (Figure 2-1).[8,9] There is also evidence that other factors, such as cytokines, nitric oxide, and the vasoconstrictor endothelin, may play a role in the pathogenesis of HF.

■ Other Pathophysiologic Considerations in HF

Myocardial Ischemia and Infarction

- The predominant cause of LV systolic dysfunction is myocardial infarction or ischemia or both. A demonstration of viability in akinetic or hypokinetic myocardium raises the possibility that the dysfunctional myocardial tissue may improve from revascularization.
- Severely restricted coronary blood flow may result in myocardial tissue that is unable to contract, although it does remain viable, at least for a period of time. This has been termed *hibernating myocardium*. The restoration of coronary flow restores normal contractility, whereas continued hibernation may ultimately lead to cell death.
- An important issue in HF is whether revascularization might substantially improve LV systolic function in patients with significant areas of hibernation.

Mitral Regurgitation

- LV remodeling results in a more globular shaped heart, which affects the geometric relation between the papillary muscles and the mitral leaflets, causing restricted opening and increased tethering of the leaflets and distortion of the mitral apparatus. Dilatation of the annulus develops as a result of increasing LV or atrial size or as a result of regional abnormalities caused by myocardial infarction. The presence of mitral regurgitation results in an increasing volume overload on the left ventricle that further contributes to remodeling, the progression of disease, and the onset of symptoms. Correction of mitral regurgitation has become an appropriate focus of therapy.

Atrial Fibrillation

- There are data that suggest a potentially important role of atrial fibrillation (AF) in the progression of HF. Studies have found that the development of AF is associated with an increased risk of hospitalization because of worsening HF. AF may also bring about ventricular systolic dysfunction by causing tachycardia-mediated cardiomyopathy.

Bilateral Renal Artery Stenosis

- The association of HF with bilateral renovascular disease is well recognized. Acute or "flash" pulmonary edema is most commonly described, but chronic HF can also occur.[10] HF develops when the kidneys, supplied by stenotic renal arteries, fail to mount a pressure natriuresis to high arterial pressure. The syndrome is therefore characterized by fluid retention rather than ventricular failure. Clinical clues include the association of cardiac and renal failure with hypertension, widespread vascular disease, the inequality of renal size (1.5 cm or greater difference) on ultrasonography, and a reversible increase in serum creatinine concentrations after taking an angiotensin-converting enzyme (ACE) inhibitor. A proportion of patients with this clinical syndrome may be cured by renal revascularization.

■ Diastolic HF

- Patients with isolated diastolic HF have pathophysiologic characteristics that are similar to those of patients with typical systolic HF, though they are less severe, including markedly reduced exercise capacity, neuroendocrine activation, and impaired quality of life.[11]

■ Sodium and Water Retention

- The abnormal activation of several homeostatic hormonal systems contribute to sodium and water retention in HF. This includes the activation of the sympathetic nervous and renin-angiotensin systems, increased release of

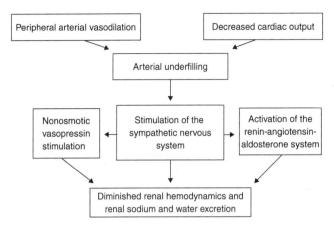

Figure 2.3: Depicted is the sequence of events in which peripheral arterial vasodilation or decreased cardiac output results in arterial underfilling, with subsequent renal sodium and water retention. Adapted from: Cadnapaphornchai MA, Gurevich AK, Weinberger HD, Schrier RW. Pathophysiology of sodium and water retention in heart failure. *Cardiology.* 2001;96:122-131.

endothelin and vasopressin, and resistance to natriuretic peptides.[12] A schematic representation of the role of these factors is depicted in Figure 2-3.

■ Mechanisms Underlying Symptoms in HF

- There is a poor relation between the symptoms of HF and hemodynamic derangements, such as cardiac output and left-sided filling pressures.[13–15]

Dyspnea

- Shortness of breath may be caused by interstitial lung edema but appears to be also related to the following:
  - Skeletal muscle structure, bulk, exercise capacity, blood flow, and intrinsic metabolic activity
  - Ventilation–perfusion mismatch in the lung

Fatigue

- Mechanisms underlying the generation of fatigue in chronic HF are complex. There is evidence implicating the following:
  - Abnormalities in muscle histology, metabolism, and quantity, along with endothelial dysfunction
  - Muscle inflammation (as recent data suggest)
  - Decreased systemic blood pressures

■ References

1.   Hunt SA, Baker DW, Chin MH, et al. ACC/AHA guidelines for the evaluation and management of chronic heart failure in the adult: executive summary. *Circulation*. 2001; 104:2996-3007.

2.   Sutton MG, Sharpe N. Left ventricular remodeling after myocardial infarction: pathophysiology and therapy. *Circulation*. 2000;101:2981-2988.

3.   Packer M. New concepts in the pathophysiology of heart failure: beneficial and deleterious interaction of endogenous haemodynamic and neurohormonal mechanisms. *J Intern Med*. 1996;239:327-333.

4.   Benedict CR, Shelton B, Johnstone DE, et al. Prognostic significance of plasma norepinephrine in patients with asymptomatic left ventricular dysfunction. SOLVD Investigators. *Circulation*. 1996;94:690-697.

5.   Rundqvist B, Elam M, Bergmann-Sverrisdottir Y, Eisenhofer G, Friberg P. Increased cardiac adrenergic drive precedes generalized sympathetic activation in human heart failure. *Circulation*. 1997;95:169-175.

6.   Packer M. Neurohumoral interactions and adaptations in congestive heart failure. *Circulation*. 1988;77:721-730.

7.   Dzau VJ. Tissue renin-angiotensin system in myocardial hypertrophy and failure. *Arch Intern Med*. 1993; 153:937-942.

8.   Wagoner LE, Walsh RA. The cellular pathophysiology of progression to heart failure. *Curr Opin Cardiol*. 1996; 11:237-244.

9.   Katz AM. The cardiomyopathy of overload: an unnatural growth response in the hypertrophied heart. *Ann Intern Med*. 1994;121:363-371.

10. Diamond JR. Flash pulmonary edema and the diagnostic suspicion of occult renal artery stenosis. *Am J Kidney Dis.* 1993;21:328-330.
11. Kitzman DW, Little WC, Brubaker PH, et al. Pathophysiological characterization of isolated diastolic heart failure in comparison to systolic heart failure. *JAMA.* 2002;288:2144-2150.
12. Cadnapaphornchai MA, Gurevich AK, Weinberger HD, Schrier RW. Pathophysiology of sodium and water retention in heart failure. *Cardiology.* 2001;96:122-131.
13. Clark AL, Poole-Wilson PA, Coats AJ. Exercise limitation in chronic heart failure: central role of the periphery. *J Am Coll Cardiol.* 1996;28:1092-1102.
14. Piepoli M, Clark AL, Volterrani M, Adamopoulos S, Sleight P, Coats AJ. Contribution of muscle afferents to the hemodynamic, autonomic, and ventilatory responses to exercise in patients with chronic heart failure: effects of physical training. *Circulation.* 1996;93:940-952.
15. Drexler H, Coats AJ. Explaining fatigue in congestive heart failure. *Annu Rev Med.* 1996;47:241-256.

Clinical Presentation of HF

■ Introduction

- The onset and severity of the symptoms of HF are variable and depend significantly on the nature of the underlying cardiac disease and the rate at which the syndrome develops. A large proportion of patients with damaged or dysfunctional hearts may remain without symptoms for months to years (stage B).
  - This, in part, may be caused by the slow transition from abnormalities of the LV chamber to systolic and diastolic myocardial dysfunction in some patients.
- Symptoms of acute HF often result from the sudden reduction in cardiac output and pulmonary congestion and are rarely accompanied by peripheral edema.

■ Symptoms and Physical Signs of Chronic HF

Dyspnea and Related Symptoms

- *Dyspnea* is defined as an exaggerated, uncomfortable awareness of breathing and may be manifested during moderate to severe physical activity in patients experiencing the early stages of HF. In patients with advanced disease, dyspnea may be present after mild exertion or even at rest.

  Patients describe these sensations in various ways:
    "air does not go all the way down"
    "shortness of breath"
    "short-windedness"
    "heavy or laboured breathing"
    "smothering feeling or tightness or tiredness in the chest"
    "choking sensation"

- *Orthopnea* is defined as breathlessness that develops in the recumbent position and is relieved by sitting upright or standing. Patients often state that they have to sleep on three or more pillows to feel comfortable at night. Dyspnea in the recumbent position is usually a later and more advanced manifestation of HF than exertional dyspnea. Orthopnea may become so severe that patients cannot lie down at all and must spend the entire night in a sitting position.

- *Paroxysmal nocturnal dyspnea (PND)* usually begins 2 to 4 hours after the onset of sleep and is associated with marked dyspnea followed by coughing, wheezing, and sweating. As with orthopnea, sitting bolt upright or getting out of bed usually relieves this symptom.

- Orthopnea and PND usually reflect varying degrees of pulmonary congestion.

- *Cheyne-Stokes respiration* is defined as periodic respiration or cyclic respiration characterized by periods of apnea followed by hyperventilation. This cyclical breathing pattern is often reported by family members of patients with advanced HF and probably reflects cerebral hypoperfusion.

Fatigue, Weakness, and Reduction in Exercise Capacity

- Although not specific to HF, fatigue and impaired exercise capacity are prominent symptoms in patients with chronic HF and add to a poor quality of life.

Fluid Retention

- Fluid retention heralds the onset of the congestive phase of HF, which may be manifested by peripheral edema, hepatomegaly, ascites, and increased circulating blood volume with elevated jugular venous distension pressures.

  - Patients may report hypochondrial tenderness or a sensation of abdominal fullness. This often results from hepatic congestion and distension of the hepatic capsule. With severe hepatic congestion, the patient may complain of nausea and anorexia in addition to upper abdominal discomfort.

Other Symptoms

- *Nocturia*: This is largely caused by the improved renal perfusion in the recumbent position at night.
- *Neurological symptoms*: Elderly patients with HF may initially present with a number of neurological symptoms, including confusion, headaches, insomnia, bad dreams, anxiety, disorientation, and impaired memory. In addition, many patients with HF may be depressed.
- *Erectile dysfunction*: This is a common and underappreciated problem for these patients and can be caused by HF itself or the medications that have been prescribed to treat it.
- Patients with less severe degrees of HF may be asymptomatic or only have mild symptoms. These may include fatigue or dyspnea during ordinary physical activity. There may be an absence of symptoms at rest.

Physical Findings

Introduction

- Many findings are associated with HF, and a wide range exists in clinicians' abilities to detect these findings. The most reliable findings for detecting increased filling pressure are jugular venous distension and radiographic vascular redistribution. The most predictive finding for detecting systolic dysfunction is an abnormal apical impulse.

General Appearance

- Physical signs vary according to the severity of HF and the predominant hemodynamic abnormality.
  - Patients with milder forms of HF often do not have any distinctive physical findings to point to the diagnosis of HF.
  - Patients with more severe HF may present with tachypnea at rest, tachycardia, and a cold and cyanotic periphery. The degree of peripheral hypoperfusion may be so advanced that the skin over the lower extremities becomes mottled (livido reticularis).

Blood Pressure and Pulse

- A diminished pulse pressure that is consistent with a reduced stroke volume and a slightly elevated diastolic arterial pressure caused by generalized vasoconstriction are often found in patients with advanced HF.
  - *Pulsus alternans* describes a strong or normal pulse that alternates with a weak pulse during normal sinus rhythm. This physical finding is relatively rare, but, when present, it is a sign of severe HF.
  - *Pulsus paradoxus* describes an expected decrease (up to 10 mm Hg) in systolic arterial pressure during inspiration that is accentuated (usually greater than 14 mm Hg). The peripheral pulse may disappear completely during inspiration in patients with pericardial tamponade. This finding has also been documented in advanced right and left ventricular dysfunction, pulmonary embolus, asthma, and right ventricular (RV) infarction.

Evidence of Increased Filling Pressures

- *Jugular venous distension*: This is found when marked right-sided congestion is present, the jugular venous pressure is elevated, the hepatojugular reflux test is positive, and the liver is enlarged.
  - The hepatojugular reflux test, defined as the increase in venous pressure in response to 15 seconds of sustained abdominal compression, suggests decreased RV compliance.
  - Elevated jugular venous distension is highly suggestive of increased left heart pressures.[1]
  - *Kussmaul's sign* is a lack of decline in jugular venous pressure during inspiration. On occasion, the jugular venous pressure increases during inspiration. This physical finding has been described in constrictive pericarditis. It has also been observed in advanced RV dysfunction.
- *Pulmonary rales*: Inspiratory, crepitant rales over the lung bases occur commonly in patients with HF and elevated pulmonary venous and capillary pressures. Rales and

wheezing may be heard widely over both lung fields in patients with pulmonary congestion. The absence of rales does not imply that the pulmonary venous pressures are not elevated. This is, in part, caused by increased and effective lymphatic drainage of alveolar fluid.

- *Pleural effusion and ascites*: Pleural effusion is more frequent in the right pleural cavity than in the left. Ascites is rarely found in moderate HF; it is most commonly found in patients with tricuspid valve disease and constrictive pericarditis.
- *Hepatomegaly*: An enlarged, tender, pulsating liver also accompanies systemic venous congestion.
- *Lower extremity edema*: This is usually evident in both legs, particularly in the pretibial region and ankles in ambulatory patients. Ankle swelling is often most prominent in the evening. Sacral edema can be detected in patients who are bed-ridden.

Cardiac Examination

- In general, patients with predominant diastolic HF may present almost normal findings in a cardiac examination. However, in patients with advanced systolic dysfunction a third heart sound may be present, and there is often a laterally displaced apex beat.[2–5] A murmur of mitral regurgitation can be heard when the left ventricle is markedly enlarged, and a tricuspid regurgitation murmur can be heard when the right ventricle is volume or pressure overloaded.
  - Among patients with HF, an elevated jugular venous pressure and a third heart sound are each independently associated with adverse outcomes, including the progression of HF.

■ Symptoms and Physical Signs of Acute HF

- The symptoms of acute pulmonary edema are more disabling than the orthopnea and paroxysmal nocturnal dyspnea experienced in chronic HF.
- In pulmonary edema, the development of severe pulmonary capillary hypertension is more rapid. Patients

typically experience a sudden, overwhelming sensation of suffocation and air hunger.

- Extreme anxiety, cough, expectoration of a pink frothy liquid, and a sensation of drowning invariably accompany this sensation. The patient often sits bolt upright, is unable to speak in full sentences, and may thrash about.
- The respiratory rate is increased, the alae nasi are dilated, and the intercostal spaces and supraclavicular fossae are retracted. Respiration is often noisy, and there may be audible inspiratory and expiratory gurgling sounds.
- An ominous sign is obtundation, which may be a sign of severe hypoxemia. Sweating is profuse, and the skin tends to be cool, ashen and cyanotic, reflecting a low cardiac output and increased sympathetic outflow.

- The blood pressure and pulse rate are most often elevated by an increased adrenergic drive. When the blood pressure is found to be markedly elevated, it is more likely to be the cause or an important contributing factor of pulmonary edema rather than the consequence of the condition.
- Auscultation of the lungs usually reveals coarse airway sounds bilaterally with rhonchi, wheezes, and moist, fine crepitant rales that are detected first at the lung bases but then upward to the apices as the lung edema worsens.
- The physical findings on examination of the heart are dependent on whether pulmonary edema is the result of cardiogenic or noncardiogenic causes; when it is cardiogenic in origin, the clinical findings reflect the underlying cardiac pathology.
- Cardiac auscultation may be difficult in the acute situation, but third and fourth heart sounds may be appreciated. The murmurs of mitral and aortic regurgitation and the systolic murmur of ischemic septal rupture may be audible, but detection requires a careful and skillful auscultator.
- An aortic outflow murmur with an absent first component of the second heart sound may be indicative of aor-

tic stenosis as the cause of HF. It should be recognized, though, that in the setting of a low cardiac output, this murmur may be greatly diminished or even absent.

■ References

1. Drazner MH, Rame JE, Stevenson LW, Dries DL. Prognostic importance of elevated jugular venous pressure and a third heart sound in patients with heart failure. *N Engl J Med.* 2001;345:574-581.

2. Badgett RG, Lucey CR, Mulrow CD. Can the clinical examination diagnose left-sided heart failure in adults? *JAMA.* 1997;277:1712-1719.

3. Drazner MH, Hamilton MA, Fonarow G, Creaser J, Flavell C, Stevenson LW. Relationship between right and left-sided filling pressures in 1000 patients with advanced heart failure. *J Heart Lung Transplant.* 1999;18:1126-1132.

4. Khot UN, Jia G, Moliterno DJ, et al. Prognostic importance of physical examination for heart failure in non-ST-elevation acute coronary syndromes: the enduring value of Killip classification. *JAMA.* 2003;290:2174-2181.

5. Weitz HH, Mangione S. In defense of the stethoscope and the bedside. *Am J Med.* 2000;108:669-671.

Assessment of Patients with HF

■ Assessment of Patients with Acute HF and Pulmonary Edema

Introduction

- It is imperative to establish the underlying cause of acute pulmonary edema so that effective treatments can be initiated. Because these patients are often hemodynamically unstable and in respiratory distress, initial stabilization is required before commencing with a diagnostic workup for the underlying cause. The following steps are suggested:

Step 1

- The most important initial step is to assess the degree of hypoxemia by obtaining an arterial blood gas analysis. When there is hypoxia (PaO_2 is less than 60 mm Hg) without hypercapnia, oxygen-enriched gas may suffice; this can be administered through nasal prongs, Venturi masks, or reservoir bag masks, depending on the severity of the gas exchange abnormality. Intubation and mechanical ventilation are usually necessary when oxygenation cannot be maintained or progressive hypercapnia is found.
- When the patient is adequately oxygenated and stable hemodynamics are ensured, the treating physician should differentiate other respiratory emergencies (e.g., asthma and pneumonia) from acute pulmonary edema as the cause of the acute respiratory syndrome.

Step 2

- As soon as it has been established that the respiratory failure is caused by pulmonary edema, the next step is to differentiate cardiogenic pulmonary edema (CPE) from noncardiogenic pulmonary edema (NCPE). This distinction can invariably be made by assessing the clinical context in which it occurs and examining the clinical data available to the clinician (see Table 4-1). The clinical data include tests that are routinely conducted on all critically ill patients, such as an electrocardiogram, a blood gas analysis, and a chest x-ray.

Table 4-1:   Differentiation of Cardiogenic Pulmonary Edema (CPE) from Noncardiogenic Pulmonary Edema (NCPE) Based on Clinical Data

	NCPE	CPE
History:	Underlying disease (pancreatitis, sepsis)	Acute cardiac event
Physical examination:	Warm periphery Bounding pulses Normal-sized heart Normal JVP No S_3 No murmurs	Cool, mottled periphery Small volume pulse Cardiomegaly Elevated JVP S_3 Systolic and diastolic murmurs
Electrocardiogram:	ECG usually normal abnormalities	ST segment and QRS complex
Chest x-ray:	Peripheral infiltrates	Perihilar infiltrates
Laboratory tests:	Normal Troponin levels BNP < 100 pg/ml	Elevated Troponin levels BNP > 100 pg/ml
Ventilation:	Requires higher FIO_2 and PEEP to oxygenate	Lower FIO_2 and PEEP to oxygenate

FIO_2, inspired oxygen concentration; JVP, jugular venous pressure; PEEP, positive end-expiratory pressure; S_3, third heart sound

Adapted from: Sibbald WJ, Cunnigham DR, Chin DN. Non-cardiac or cardiac pulmonary edema? a practical approach to clinical differentiation in critically ill patients. *Chest.* 1983;84:452-461.

- It is worthwhile to emphasize that NCPE is invariably associated with an underlying disease, which may or may not be readily apparent. The diagnosis of NCPE often depends on pretest probabilities; for example, acute respiratory distress in a patient with documented sepsis (i.e., peritonitis) or pancreatitis should raise the strong possibility that the respiratory failure is caused by NCPE. Unlike CPE, NCPE is uncommonly associated with a well-defined acute cardiac event (i.e., myocardial infarction). Subtle physical signs may also aid in differentiating NCPE from CPE. NCPE is usually a hyperdynamic illness and is clinically apparent as a warm, vasodilated periphery, whereas CPE is frequently associated with a low cardiac output, resulting in a cool, mottled periphery. The findings of a third heart sound or murmurs of aortic and mitral regurgitation and aortic stenosis are usually suggestive of a cardiogenic cause of pulmonary edema.

- Electrocardiographic ST segment changes consistent with infarction or ischemia would suggest an acute cardiac event as the cause of the pulmonary edema. Also, electrocardiographic evidence of LV strain, left bundle branch block, or other abnormalities of the QRS complex may be indicative of an underlying cardiac pathology. Unless there are major metabolic disturbances, the electrocardiogram is usually normal in patients with pure NCPE.

- In both NCPE and CPE, arterial hypoxemia is caused by changes in the ventilation–perfusion ratio and in the extent of intrapulmonary shunting. Patients with NCPE usually have a more pronounced defect in oxygenation than patients with CPE. This is largely because of the greater shunt fractions found in these patients. Thus, in the clinical setting, higher concentrations of inspired oxygen concentrations (FiO_2) and higher positive end-expiratory pressures are required to achieve acceptable oxygenation for patients with NCPE compared to CPE.

- Like other tests, the chest x-ray may be helpful to differentiate NCPE from CPE. In cases of NCPE, the alveolar and interstitial disease may show a predominant peripheral distribution, but in CPE, a perihilar distribution is more evident—often associated with Kerley's lines or pleural effusions or both. Heart size is more commonly increased in CPE than in NCPE, but the lack of cardiomegaly by no means excludes CPE. Unfortunately, in the majority of patients, the chest x-ray proves to be of little help. This is is partly because patients are often too ill to be examined by anything other than a portable unit, and films from such units are usually of suboptimal interpretive quality.

Step 3

- When the cause of pulmonary edema is clearly evident from the clinical data (i.e., myocardial infarction), no further diagnostic tests are needed. If there is still uncertainty regarding the etiology of the pulmonary edema, further diagnostic tests are appropriate.
  - A rapid assay for *B-type natriuretic peptide* (BNP) can be used to diagnose HF.[1,2] Normal levels are less than 100 pg/ml. The test has a negative predictive value of 96%, which implies that CPE can effectively be ruled out for patients in the normal range. However, it only has a positive predictive value of 90%. Elevated BNP levels are found in patients with increasing age, pulmonary hypertension, cor pulmonale, pulmonary emboli, and compensated HF. Also, BNP levels appear to be less useful in patients with renal failure. Thus, clinical judgment is still required to differentiate CPE from NCPE.
  - In the past, the placement of a pulmonary artery balloon flotation catheter was used to differentiate CPE from NCPE, but with the general availability of BNP levels and two-dimensional echocardiography, there seems to be less need for pulmonary artery catheter placement. Pulmonary artery catheterization may be more useful in guiding therapy rather than establishing the diagnosis.
  - A reasonable approach, therefore, is to obtain an echocardiogram for all patients with pulmonary edema in whom the cause of pulmonary edema is unclear.

Step 4:

- Should the etiology be unclear even after BNP levels and echocardiographic data have been obtained, the clinician may be required to attempt a diagnostic–therapeutic trial. A brief but meaningful regimen of diuretic therapy is initiated, and both subjective and objective criteria for improvement are monitored.

Step 5:

- After establishing that the cause of pulmonary edema is cardiogenic in origin and initial steps have been taken to ensure optimal oxygenation, it becomes critically important to: (1) define the underlying cardiac etiology, (2) characterize the dominant hemodynamic abnormality, and (3) identify precipitating factors.

Etiology of CPE

- Acute decompensation of systolic and diastolic LV function may occur both in the setting of chronic HF and as a new entity, for example, with extensive myocardial ischemia. Furthermore, overt HF may be evident for the first time in a previously stable, compensated patient when the intrinsic underlying myocardial process has advanced to a critical point, such as in a patient with progressive narrowing of a stenotic aortic valve or when a cardiac or noncardiac event unmasks a previously asymptomatic cardiac disease—such as pulmonary edema precipitated by atrial fibrillation in a patient with previously unrecognized mitral stenosis.
- The patient's history offers the best clue to whether there is underlying chronic heart disease, but abnormal physical signs (e.g., a murmur of aortic stenosis) or an abnormal electrocardiogram (e.g., evidence of a previous infarction) or echocardiogram (e.g., a large heart and a globally decreased LV systolic function) may provide useful information regarding the extent and acuteness of the syndrome.
- Crucial to the appropriate management of a patient with acute HF is the establishment of an underlying etiology.

The most common causes of acute HF are listed in Table 1-3. Acute, extensive myocardial infarction is probably the most frequently encountered cause of acute HF and is usually obvious from the history and the characteristic electrocardiographic changes. It should also be recognized that, in the absence of chest pain, pulmonary edema can be the first manifestation of severe coronary artery disease, especially in the elderly diabetic who is hypertensive. In a large percentage of patients, the diagnosis will be obvious from the history, physical examination, and electrocardiogram, but in some the diagnosis will not be evident. For such patients, the echocardiogram may provide invaluable information. An echocardiographic assessment of the left ventricle could establish whether there is LV systolic dysfunction, LV hypertrophy, focal wall abnormalities, ventricular septal rupture, acute valvular regurgitation, or a stenotic aortic or mitral valve. However, it should be emphasized that a normal echocardiogram does not exclude recent myocardial ischemia as a possible cause of acute HF.

Hemodynamic Abnormality

- Because an elevated LV filling pressure is a prerequisite for the extravasation of fluid into the alveolar space, all patients with CPE, by definition, will have diastolic LV dysfunction. Therefore, it is important to identify whether diastolic LV dysfunction is associated with either decreased or preserved LV systolic function. For example, patients with those forms of hypertrophic cardiomyopathy in which there is normal systolic function and markedly elevated LV diastolic pressures may not benefit from inotropic or arteriolar vasodilator drugs.
- It is often difficult to separate those with good systolic function from others by means of history, physical examination, or initial laboratory tests. Although patients with preserved systolic function are more likely to be hypertensive, this fact does not help categorize any individual patient. Further diagnostic tests are usually indicated when the clinical data do not completely define the dominant hemodynamic abnormality.

Precipitating Causes of Acute HF

■ These factors can be defined as those factors that may precipitate acute decompensation in patients with underlying cardiac disease, but are unlikely to cause cardiac decompensation in patients with normal hearts. Identifying the precipitating causes of the acute hemodynamic decompensation has obvious therapeutic implications. A list of the more common precipitating causes is shown in Table 4-2.

  • Many of the cardiac arrhythmias that can exacerbate the hemodynamic and clinical status of patients with HF are of supraventricular origin. These tachyarrhythmias reduce the time available for LV filling, an event that is particularly deleterious in patients with impaired myocardial relaxation. Moreover, tachycardia increases myocardial oxygen consumption and decreases the time available for myocardial perfusion and, thus, may exacerbate myocardial ischemia.

Table 4-2:   Precipitating Causes of Heart Failure

■ Dietary indiscretion
■ Vigorous postoperative fluid resuscitation
■ Noncompliance to medical regiment
■ Worsening renal failure
■ Anemia
■ Systemic infection
■ Pulmonary embolism
■ Myocardial ischemia
■ Tachyarrhythmias and bradyarrhythmias
■ Electrolyte disturbances
■ Hyperthyroidism and hypothyroidism
■ Cardiodepressant drugs and other drugs that may worsen heart failure:
  • Anti-inflammatory drugs:
      Steroids, nonsteroidal and anti-inflammatory agents
  • Antiarrhythmic drugs:
      Disopyramide, Flecainide, Encainide, Mexilitine, Tocainide, Procainamide, Lidocaine
  • Calcium channel blockers:
      Verapimil, Diltiazem, Nifedipine
  • β-blocking agents

- Mild ischemia that ordinarily may not have a major hemodynamic effect may precipitate acute pulmonary edema in elderly patients with LV hypertrophy caused by hypertension or in patients with compromised ventricular function (large prior myocardial infarction). Ischemia may manifest as episodes of typical angina or may occur without symptoms.
- Several commonly used medications, such as nonsteroidal anti-inflammatory drugs, the newer oral hypoglycemic agents (glitazones), certain antiarrhythmic drugs, calcium channel blocking agents and β-adrenergic blocking agents, may exacerbate the symptoms of HF in patients with severe LV systolic dysfunction.

■ Assessment and Recognition of Asymptomatic and Symptomatic LV Systolic Dysfunction

- Patients with LV systolic dysfunction present with decreased exercise tolerance or evidence of fluid retention or both. A patient may also present without symptoms, in which case LV dysfunction is incidentally discovered.
- The recognition of asymptomatic patients with LV dysfunction and those with mild to moderate HF may be difficult.
  - Many of the signs and symptoms of chronic HF may also occur in other conditions, such as obesity and chronic noncardiac diseases.[3–5] In elderly patients, the diagnosis of early or even more advanced HF may not be made because these patients often lead a fairly sedentary life as a consequence of their age and other debilitating noncardiac problems.
  - The simplest approach to this problem is to exercise a high index of suspicion when an asymptomatic patient is encountered with certain physical signs and radiologic and electrocardiographic abnormalities. The clinical findings that would alert one to suspect LV dysfunction are listed in Table 4-3.

Table 4-3:   Clinical Indicators of Asymptomatic LV Systolic and Diastolic Dysfunction

History:
- Alcohol or cocaine abuse
- Prior myocardial infarction(s)
- Previous chemotherapy
- Long-standing hypertension
- Family history of heart failure

Physical signs:
- Resting tachycardia
- Displaced apical impulse
- Third or fourth heart sound or both
- Mitral regurgitant murmur

Electrocardiographic findings:
- Evidence of extensive ischemic myocardial injury
- T-wave abnormalities or left bundle branch block or both
- New onset of atrial fibrillation or other arrhythmias

Chest x-ray:
- Increased cardiothoracic ratio
- Apical redistribution of pulmonary blood flow

- In contrast to asymptomatic LV dysfunction, the identification of moderate to severe HF is far less problematic, especially when a patient presents with the triad of *fluid retention, exertional dyspnea and fatigue,* and *evidence of structural heart disease.* The following observations, however, should be kept in mind:
  - Symptoms of fluid retention (i.e., a congested state) do not necessarily indicate HF. Many patients diagnosed as having HF on the grounds of pedal edema do not have HF.
  - Exertional dyspnea or fatigue may be caused by HF, although it could also be caused by a range of other conditions, all of which should be considered before attributing these symptoms to HF. These conditions include, among others, pulmonary embolism, pneu-

monia, chronic obstructive lung disease, asthma, pulmonary fibrosis, pleural effusion, anemia, hyperthyroidism, and musculoskeletal disorders.

- In order to overcome the lack of accuracy in diagnosing HF, various clinical criteria (e.g., Framingham criteria) have been developed to improve and standardize the recognition of this syndrome.
  - The utility of these criteria to establish the diagnosis of mild to moderate HF in the primary health care setting is questionable.
  - The simplest approach to improve the diagnostic accuracy may be correlating the typical symptoms that are associated with the HF syndrome with echocardiographic evidence of structural heart disease.
- A growing body of evidence suggests that the measurement of plasma BNP concentrations represents a useful addition to the chest x-ray, electrocardiogram, and Doppler echocardiography in the clinical assessment of patients suspected of having HF. The following guidelines are suggested[1]:
  - For new patients presenting with suspected HF in the outpatient setting, BNP testing is most useful as a "rule-out" test for HF. If the BNP is less than 100 pg/ml in untreated patients, then HF is highly unlikely.
  - If the BNP concentration is raised (100 pg/ml or greater), then there is a strong possibility that the patient has HF, for which the patient should be fully investigated. Other conditions, such as cor pulmonale, AF, and strokes, can also elevate BNP levels.
  - There are inconclusive data for the role of screening for asymptomatic LV systolic dysfunction using BNP in the general population.
  - BNP increases significantly with age and is significantly higher in women than in men, leading to age-specific and gender-specific reference ranges.[6]
- An outline of the diagnostic approach used to recognize the patients with asymptomatic and symptomatic LV dysfunction or HF of varying severity is shown in Figure 4-1.

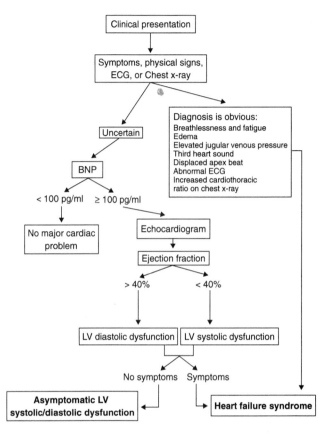

Figure 4-1: This outline represents an integrative approach to recognizing patients with asymptomatic LV dysfunction and HF. The history, physical, electrocardiographic, and chest x-ray findings are used together with echocardiographic findings, where appropriate, to diagnose asymptomatic LV dysfunction or the clinical syndrome of HF. The diagnosis of the HF syndrome may be obvious when a patient has symptoms, physical signs, and electrocardiogram (ECG) and chest x-ray findings that are consistent with HF. Under these circumstances, no further tests are needed to diagnose this condition. However, echocardiographic information may well be needed later on to define the etiology and severity of LV dysfunction. BNP levels (see main text) could be obtained when there is uncertainty about the diagnosis. Levels greater than 100 pg/ml are suggestive but not confirmative of HF. An echocardiogram would add additional information about the extent of LV systolic dysfunction (ejection fraction less than 40%) or LV diastolic dysfunction (ejection fraction greater than 40%, presence of Doppler LV filling abnormalities, or LV hypertrophy).

■ Assessment and Recognition of Asymptomatic and Symptomatic LV Diastolic Dysfunction

- The symptoms of diastolic HF are largely indistinguishable from those of HF caused by impaired systolic function.[2]
- The risk of HF increases dramatically with increasing severity of diastolic dysfunction.
- Severe diastolic dysfunction is often asymptomatic.
- Population-based studies have repeatedly demonstrated that 40% to 50% of individuals with HF have normal LVEF.
- Abnormal mitral inflow patterns obtained with Doppler echocardiography, suggesting mild or moderate or severe diastolic dysfunction, are independently predictive of the future development of HF in older asymptomatic patients.
- Asymptomatic diastolic dysfunction is essentially a Doppler echocardiographic diagnosis based on the presence of mitral inflow abnormalities.
- The diagnosis of diastolic HF can be made without the measurement of parameters that reflect LV diastolic function.[7]

■ Recognition of Specific Chronic HF Syndromes

Dominant Right-Sided HF

- Predominant right-sided HF may result from dysfunctional RV myocardium, excessive RV afterload or preload, restriction to RV filling, or a combination of these.
- The clinical signs of right-sided HF are more or less similar regardless of the etiology (Table 4-4) and are manifested by elevated filling pressures and decreased right-sided output, the extent of which depends on the rate at which the right-sided failure develops.
- An acute or recent onset of right-sided failure, secondary to RV infarction, acute severe pulmonary embolism, or cardiac tamponade, is usually characterized by elevated jugular venous pressure and a depressed cardiac output.

Table 4-4: Clinical Characteristics of Common Right-Sided Failure Syndromes

Etiology	Clinical features	Electrocardiographic findings	Echocardiographic features
Acute:			
RV infarction*	Hypotension; Kussmaul's sign	Inferior MI; ST elevation in right-sided leads	Inferior wall motion abnormality; RV dilation and decreased systolic function
Acute pulmonary embolism	Acute dyspnea; borderline hemodynamics; hypoxia	Sinus tachycardia; acute RV strain; S_1, Q_3, T_3	RV dilation and decreased systolic dysfunction; flattening of the interventricular septum
Cardiac tamponade	Venous pulse: prominent x descent; hypotension; pulsus paradoxus	Sinus tachycardia; low voltage and varies with respiration	Moderate to large pericardial effusion; RV, RA, and LA collapse
Chronic:			
Cor pulmonale* (COPD and restrictive lung disease, PTED, PPH, and Eisenmenger's syndrome)	History: smoking, recurrent emboli, congenital disease; cyanosis; plethora TR murmur; loud P_2	Right axis; RV strain; p-pulmonale	RV dilation and decreased systolic dysfunction; flattening of the interventricular septum
LV systolic dysfunction*	LV apex displaced S_3; MR murmur; Previous MI(s)	LBBB; diffuse T-wave abnormalities	Dilated, poorly contractile LV; varying degrees of MR; restrictive mitral filling pattern

Table 4-4: continued

Etiology	Clinical features	Electrocardiographic findings	Echocardiographic features
Mitral valve disease	Characteristic murmurs; loud P_2	RV strain; p-mitrale	Stenotic or regurgitant mitral valve; large LA; dilated RV
Tricuspid regurgitation (IV drug abuse)	Venous pulse; prominent CV wave	RA enlargement	Abnormal tricuspid valve; dilated RA and RV; normal RV systolic function
Constrictive pericarditis	Prominent x and y descents; Kussmaul's sign; pericardial knock; x-ray: calcified pericardium	Diffuse T-wave inversion	Small RV and LV, but large atria; restrictive mitral filling pattern; abnormal hepatic vein flow

This table highlights clinical aspects that may be useful in identifying the specific cause of predominant right-sided failure. It is assumed that all patients will present varying degrees of jugular venous distension and peripheral edema. Asterisks (*) indicate the most common causes of right-sided failure. COPD, chronic obstructive pulmonary disease; LA, left atrial; LBBB, left bundle branch block; LV, left ventricular; LVH, left ventricular hypertrophy; MI, myocardial infarction; MR, mitral regurgitation; P_2, pulmonary component of the second heart sound; PPH, primary pulmonary hypertension; PTED, pulmonary thromboembolic disease; RA, right atrial; RV, right ventricular; S_3, third heart sound; TR, tricuspid regurgitation.

- Because of the acute nature of these conditions, they are, as a rule, not associated with a generalized edematous state. In contrast, marked fluid retention as manifested by peripheral edema, visceromegaly, and ascites is more consistent with chronic right-sided failure.
- The most common cause of right-sided failure is advanced LV systolic dysfunction, and the second most common cause is cor pulmonale that is secondary to chronic lung disease.
- The recognition of certain causes of right-sided failure is important, because the management differs considerably from that of predominant left-sided failure.
  - For example, the treatment of right-sided failure that is secondary to chronic obstructive pulmonary disease should be directed towards maximizing oxygenation, whereas right-sided failure caused by LV dysfunction is usually managed by diuretics, ACE inhibitors, digitalis, and afterload-reducing agents.

High-Output HF

- HF may be characterized by a high-output state resulting from decreased peripheral resistance, and it is clinically manifested by tachycardia, bounding pulses, warm periphery, pistol-shot femoral pulses, a third heart sound, and varying degrees of fluid retention.
- Identifying this syndrome is important, because many of the conditions associated with high-output HF are reversible (Table 4-5).
- Certain conditions associated with increased cardiac output, such as anemia, rarely cause HF, and when failure is apparent, it is likely that abnormal hemodynamic factors are superimposed on an underlying cardiac abnormality, such as valvular heart disease or myocardial dysfunction.

■ Etiologic Considerations of Chronic HF

- Once there is reasonable certainty that the clinical findings are consistent with HF, further diagnostic testing is indicated to accomplish the following:
  - Establish the primary cardiac pathology

Table 4-5: High Output Heart Failure Syndromes: Clinical Characteristics, Pathophysiologic Mechanisms, and Diagnostic Tests

Etiology	Clinical features	Pathophysiologic mechanisms	Diagnostic tests
Chronic anemia	Pale appearance (When failure is present, search for underlying cardiac pathology.)	Decreased O_2 carrying capacity, blood viscosity, and peripheral vascular resistance, with augmented venous return	Markedly decreased hemoglobin and hematocrit
Arteriovenous fistula or other conditions that produce arteriovenous shunting (Paget's disease and hepatic disease)	Continuous murmur over fistula or arteriovenous malformation; Branham's sign*	Decreased peripheral vascular resistance and increased preload	Ultrasound or angiography or both
Beriberi	Alcohol abuse; peripheral neuritis	Thiamine deficiency leading to autonomic dysfunction; other mechanisms as listed above	Low blood thiamine levels and erythrocyte transketolase activity
Hyperthyroidism	Atrial arrhythmias; enlarged thyroid; elderly patient; (Seek underlying cardiac disease.)	Decreased peripheral vascular resistance and increased preload	Thyroid function tests

*Branham's sign: slowing of the heart after manual compression of the fistula.

- Evaluate the extent of extracardiac (e.g., renal) involvement
- Identify disease states that are amenable to specific interventions
- Evaluate and recognize factors that are likely to have contributed or will conceivably contribute to the development and progression of HF

■ The Agency for Health Care Policy and Research and the American College of Cardiology/American Heart Association Task Force on the evaluation and management of HF have made several recommendations for diagnostic testing in patients with stable HF caused by LV systolic dysfunction (Table 4-6).[8]

- These recommendations are divided into those tests that should be conducted routinely in all patients with a recent onset of HF as well as the tests that may be helpful for selected patients.

■ Figure 4-2 provides a logical and cost-effective outline of the diagnostic steps that are necessary to adequately assess patients that present with a recent onset of HF. This approach relies on the clinical judgment of the physician and the physician's ability to integrate clinical data with the echocardiographic findings.

■ An important part of the diagnostic workup in patients with a recent onset of HF is the identification of reversible causes of HF. Table 4-7 lists disease entities that may be associated with reversible myocardial dysfunction.

■ Common Errors in the Diagnosis and Evaluation of HF

■ The Agency for Health Care Policy and Research has identified several aspects of the diagnosis and evaluation of HF patients in the community that are not optimal.[8] These include the following:

- Patients with symptoms suggestive of HF are often not thoroughly evaluated to rule out noncardiac causes before treatment for HF is started.
- Symptoms of HF may be attributed to chronic lung disease and may be treated inappropriately.

Table 4-6: Recommended Diagnostic and Other Tests for the Evaluation of Heart Failure

Test/Procedure	AHCPR		ACC/AHA		Rationale
	All pts	Selected pts	All pts	Selected pts	*(narrow differential diagnosis for HF and/or identification of factors that contribute to HF)*
Laboratory tests:					
CBC	+	–	+	–	Detect anemia, a contributing factor to HF
Electrolytes	+	–	+	–	Detect electrolyte disturbances
Urea / Cr	+	–	+	–	Assess renal function; guide to treatment
Albumin	+	–	+	–	Exclude hypoalbuminemia as a cause of edema
LFTs	+	–	+	–	Assess liver function
Ca^{++}/Mg^{++}/PO$^-_4$	–	+	+	–	Detect electrolyte disturbances
Urinalysis	+	–	+	–	Exclude nephrotic syndrome
T$_4$/TSH	–	+	–	+	Detect occult hyperthyroidism in the elderly and in patients with atrial fibrillation
Other routine tests:					
ECG, Chest x-ray	+	–	+	–	Establish recent infarction; detect pneumonia
Echo-Doppler	+	–	+	–	Detect valvular and wall motion abnormalities
Stress test with imaging	–	+	–	+	Assess extent of ischemia
Ambulatory ECG	–	+	–	+	Assess cause of syncope
Endomyocardial biopsy	–	–	–	+	Diagnose infiltrative disorders (i.e., hemochromatosis)
Measurement of ex. capacity	–	+	–	+	Assess functional status

Recommended routine diagnostic tests for patients (pts) with stable heart failure according to the Agency for Health Care Policy and Research (ACHPR) and the American College of Cardiology/American Heart Association (ACC/AHA) Task Force on Evaluation and Management of Heart Failure. A plus sign (+) indicates tests that should routinely be conducted; a negative sign (–) indicates tests that should not routinely be conducted; CBC, complete blood count; Cr, creatinine; ECG, electrocardiogram; ex., exercise; HF, heart failure; LFTs, liver function tests; T$_4$, thyroxine; TSH, thyroid-stimulating hormone.

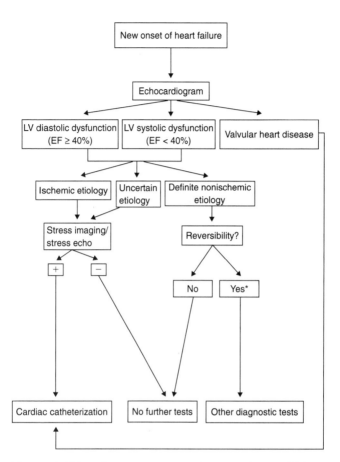

Figure 4-2: This outline represents a stepwise approach to establishing the etiology of the underlying cardiac pathology of HF and identifying reversible and contributing factors. Once there is certainty about the diagnosis of the clinical syndrome of HF, the next step is to characterize the predominant hemodynamic abnormality. Echocardiography identifies whether HF is caused by LV systolic dysfunction (ejection fraction less than 40%) or LV diastolic dysfunction (ejection fraction greater than 40%) or valvular heart disease (often associated with LV systolic and diastolic dysfunction).

The next step is to rule out an ischemic etiology. When it is unclear whether ischemia caused or contributed to LV dysfunction (uncertain etiology), stress imaging (thallium scintigraphy/pharmacologic stress testing) or stress echo may help clarify this issue.

Further testing is intended to establish whether LV dysfunction can be completely or partially reversed. Cardiac catheterization is indicated when reversible ischemia is suspected or demonstrated by noninvasive tests. *Reversible causes of a nonischemic cardiomyopathy should be excluded (e.g., a patient with suspected hemochromatosis will require iron studies).

Table 4-7: Reversible Myocardial Dysfunction: Causes, Clinical Features, and Treatment

Etiology	Clinical features	Treatment
Ischemic	Angina, ischemic ECG, positive stress imaging scans	Revascularization
Toxins:		
Alcohol	History of alcoholism, ↑MVC, ↑GGT	Abstinence
Anthracyclines	Recent chemotherapy	Termination of treatment
Cocaine	Use of cocaine, hyperadrenergic state	Abstinence
Endotoxic sepsis	Gram negative sepsis	Transient; treat bacteremia
Infections:		
Viral	Recent viral illness, myopericarditis	Supportive treatment only
Lyme disease	Conduction abn., skin and joint involvement	Usually resolves within 6 months
Toxoplasmosis	AIDS, lymphadenopathy	Antibiotics
Mycoplasma	Pneumonia, cold, agglutinins	Antibiotics
Metabolic:		
Hypocalcemia	Hypoparathyroidism, ↑Q-T interval	Calcium and parathyroid hormone
Hypophosphatemia	Alcoholism, hyperalimentation, recovery of DKA	Phosphate
Uremia	Renal failure	Dialysis

Endocrinopathies:		
Hyperthyroidism	Hyperthyroid state, elderly patient	Antithyroid drugs, I₂ or surgery
Pheochromocytoma	Hyperadrenergic state, hypertension	Tumor excision
Acromegaly	Typical acromegalic features	Surgery or radiation
Infiltrative disorders:		
Hemochromatosis	Bronze diabetic, cirrhosis, ↑serum ferritin	Chelation therapy, phlebotomy
Sarcoid	Skin and lung manifestations, conduction abn.	Steroids
Nutritional deficiencies:		
Beriberi	Alcohol abuse, polyneuropathy	Thiamine
Carnitine deficiency	Inherited progressive skeletal myopathy	Carnitine
Selenium	Occurs mainly in China	Selenium
Miscellaneous:		
Tachycardia-induced CMO	Incessant SVT or AF with ↑ ventricular response	ß-blockers, ablation
Peripartum CMO	Occurs within 6 months of delivery	Spontaneous recovery

Abn, abnormalities; AF, atrial fibrillation; CMO, cardiomyopathy; ECG, electrocardiogram; GGT, gamma glutamyl transferase; MCV, mean corpuscular volume; SVT, supraventricular tachycardia; ↑, increased.

- Reversible causes of HF are not always identified, or, when identified, they may be undertreated.
- Patients with peripheral edema may be inappropriately labeled as having HF when there is, in fact, another cause for edema.
- An initial measurement of LV function is not always obtained.
- Concurrent angina or other evidence of ischemia is not always properly evaluated.

■ Evaluation of Refractory HF

- The evaluation of patients that remain symptomatic despite optimal treatment requires an assessment of whether other conditions or contributing factors are

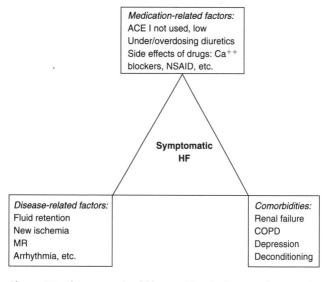

Figure 4-3: Three areas should be considered when a patient remains symptomatic after optimal medical treatment: (1) disease-related factors (e.g., worsening ischemia, a new onset of mitral regurgitation [MR], or atrial fibrillation), (2) comorbidities (e.g., sleep apnea, renal failure, or exacerbation of chronic obstructive pulmonary disease [COPD], and (3) medication-related factors (e.g., inadequate diuretic doses, over diuresis, calcium blockers, or nonsteroidal anti-inflammatory drugs [NSAID]).

responsible for the refractory symptoms before further treatment is initiated. Figure 4-3 highlights the factors that should be considered.

■ Severity and Prognosis of HF

- An important component of the initial evaluation is to assess the severity of HF, because this will determine both the overall prognosis and the initial and long-term treatment strategies.
- Assessment of the severity further enables one to identify high-risk patients who might derive benefit from more aggressive medical or surgical therapy. In addition, it is useful to document the extent of functional impairment during the first encounter with the patient so that it may be used as a reference for subsequent assessments.
- The severity of symptoms is an important indicator of overall morbidity and mortality. The most widely utilized symptom scale is the New York Heart Association (NYHA) functional classification (Table 4-8), but the accuracy and reproducibility is limited. For example, the NYHA classification is not predictive of the degree of LV dysfunction or of exercise capacity.

Table 4-8: New York Heart Association Classification of Heart Failure

Class I	*No limitations:* Ordinary physical activity does not cause undue fatigue, dyspnea, or palpitation.
Class II	*Slight limitation of physical activity:* Patients are comfortable at rest, but ordinary physical activities lead to fatigue, shortness of breath, or palpitations.
Class III	*Marked limitation of physical activity:* Although patients are comfortable at rest, less than ordinary activity will lead to symptoms.
Class IV	*Inability to engage in any physical activity without discomfort:* Symptoms are present at rest.

Table 4-9: Factors that Predict Survival in Patients with Heart Failure

Factors	Comments
Etiology of HF: Ischemic vs. nonischemic Cause of nonischemic myopathy	Ischemic LV dysfunction is associated with a higher mortality than nonischemic LV dysfunction. HIV, infiltrative (amyloid), and Doxorubicin-related cardiomyopathies have worse prognoses than idiopathic and postpartum cardiomyopathy.
Subtypes of HF: Systolic vs. diastolic HF Systolic and diastolic dysfunction	Systolic dysfunction is associated with a worse long-term prognosis than diastolic dysfunction. Diastolic dysfunction that is coexistent with impaired systolic function worsens survival.
Demographic factors: Age Race	Risk of death in patients 64 years and older at 1 year is 1.5 times greater than that of those younger than 64 years. African-Americans have about 1.5 to 2.0 times the mortality risk when diagnosed with heart failure than whites.
Hemodynamic parameters: LV ejection fraction RV ejection fraction	The mortality risk related to depressed ejection fraction is markedly increased for each increment of the ejection fraction under 30%. RV ejection fraction, as measured by radionucleotide techniques, appears to be directly related to survival in patients with NYHA class II and IV heart failure.
Symptoms and functional impairment: NYHA classification	Survival is inversely related to NYHA class.

Peak O_2 consumption 6-minute walk test	With similar ejection fractions, peak O_2 consumption of less than 14 ml/kg/min predicts a high 1-year mortality. A total distance of less than 305 m was associated with an annual mortality rate of 11% vs. 4% in patients who could walk for more than 443 m.
Electrolytes and neurohumoral factors: Sodium	A sodium concentration of less than 130 mEq/L was shown to be associated with a survival rate of less than 20% compared to nearly 50% for those with a sodium level of over 130 mEq/L.
BNP and Troponin I	Marked elevations in BNP and troponin I correlate with hemodynamic severity and prognosis in HF.
Arrhythmias: Nonsustained ventricular tachycardia (NSVT)	Two studies have shown prospectively that NSVT is an independent risk factor for sudden death in patients with heart failure.
Comorbid conditions associated with increased mortality: Hepatic dysfunction Renal dysfunction Hypertension Diabetes Pulmonary hypertension Cardiac cachexia Sleep apnea	

- Several tools, of which the *Minnesota Living with Heart Failure Questionnaire* is the most widely used, have been developed to measure the quality of life of HF patients.[9] These tools are more useful in research settings than in the clinical management of patients.

- Exercise testing with a measurement of peak oxygen consumption is widely accepted as the best index of the severity of HF.[10] Maximum oxygen consumption not only has been shown to be an independent predictor of mortality in large treatment trials but it has become a valuable tool in determining the need and timing of cardiac transplantation. However, such testing is not routinely available in an outpatient setting, and it is probably not needed for the vast majority of patients.

- A useful and simple measure of the severity of HF is the 6-minute walk test. This test can be safely conducted in the outpatient setting and has been shown in clinical trials to predict mortality and morbidity.[11,12]

■ Factors That Predict Survival in Patients with HF

- In addition to addressing the functional disability of patients with HF, several factors appear to be predictive of increased mortality. Table 4-9 provides a list of the cardiac and noncardiac factors that affect survival.

■ References

1. Cowie MR, Jourdain P, Maisel A, et al. Clinical applications of B-type natriuretic peptide (BNP) testing. *Eur Heart J.* 2003;19:1710-1718.

2: McCullough PA, Nowak RM, McCord J, et al. B-type natriuretic peptide and clinical judgment in emergency diagnosis of heart failure: analysis from Breathing Not Properly (BNP) multinational study. *Circulation.* 2002;106:416-422.

3. Mattleman SJ, Hakki AH, Iskandrian AS, Segal BL, Kane SA. Reliability of bedside evaluation in determining left ventricular function: correlation with left ventricular ejection fraction determined by ventriculography. *J Am Coll Cardiol.* 1983;1:417-420.

4. Remes J, Miettinen H, Reunanen A, Pyörälä K. Validity of clinical diagnosis of heart failure in primary health care. *Eur Heart J*. 1991;12:315-321.

5. Ikram H. Identifying the patient with heart failure. *J Int Med Res*. 1995;23:139-153.

6. Redfield MM, Rodeheffer RJ, Jacobsen SJ, Mahoney DW, Bailey KR, Burnett JC Jr. Plasma brain natriuretic peptide concentration: impact of age and gender. *J Am Coll Cardiol*. 2002;40:976-982.

7. Redfield MM, Jacobsen SJ, Burnett JC Jr, Mahoney DW, Bailey KR, Rodeheffer RJ. Burden of systolic and diastolic ventricular dysfunction in the community: appreciating the scope of the heart failure epidemic. *JAMA*. 2003;289: 194-202.

8. Konstam M, Dracup K, Baker D, et al. *Heart Failure: Evaluation and Care of Patients with Left Ventricular Systolic Dysfunction*. Rockville, MD: Agency for Health Care Policy and Research and the National Heart, Lung, and Blood Institute, Public Health Service, US Department of Health and Human Services; June 1994. Clinical Practice Guideline, No. 11 (amended) AHCPR publication 94-0612.

9. Rector TS, Cohn JN, for the Pimobendan Multicenter Research Group. Assessment of patient outcome with the Minnesota Living with Heart Failure questionnaire: reliability and validity during a randomized, double-blind, placebo-controlled trial of pimobendan. *Am Heart J*. 1992;124:1017-1025.

10. Mancini DM, Eisen H, Kussmaul W, Mull R, Edmunds LH Jr, Wilson JR. Value of peak exercise oxygen consumption for optimal timing of cardiac transplantation in ambulatory patients with heart failure. *Circulation*. 1991;83: 778-786.

11. Lipkin DP, Scriven AJ, Crake T, Poole-Wilson PA. Six minute walking test for assessing exercise capacity in chronic heart failure. *Br Med J*. 1986;292:653-655.

12. Bittner V, Weiner DH, Yusuf S, et al. Prediction of mortality and morbidity with a 6-minute walk test in patients with left ventricular dysfunction. SOLVD Investigators. *JAMA*. 1993;270:1702-1707.

Management of Patients with HF

■ Goals of Therapy

- The principal objectives of treatment for patients with HF are to enhance quality and duration of life and to attenuate, prevent, or actually reverse the progression of LV dysfunction.
- The relative importance of these therapeutic goals will vary depending on the clinical stage of HF. As HF progresses from the asymptomatic to the severe state, the focus of management shifts from interventions that halt or reverse LV dysfunction to treatments that are also aimed at relieving symptoms and preventing complications.
- To achieve these objectives, the management of HF is based on three goals:
  - Removal and amelioration of the underlying cause
  - Removal and treatment of the precipitating causes
  - Containment of the HF syndrome

■ Management of Acute HF and Pulmonary Edema

- The management of patients with CPE is primarily aimed at restoring the perfusion of vital organs and relieving pulmonary congestion. In hemodynamic terms, the intention is to increase cardiac output and lower LV filling pressure and, at the same time, ensure adequate coronary perfusion.

General Measures

- Several general measures are advisable for most patients with pulmonary congestion. Bed rest should be enforced.

Patients feel most comfortable in the semiupright position with legs dependent. Special attention should be devoted to maintaining adequate oxygenation. In most patients with CPE, arterial hypoxemia can be reversed by oxygen administration with nasal prongs or a Venturi mask. If this is not effective, continuous positive airway pressure can be administered safely by mask.

- Such treatment improves gas exchange, decreases circulatory stress, decreases respiratory work, and may reduce the need for ventilator treatment. Arterial blood gasses should be determined and endotracheal intubation should be considered if the arterial PO_2 cannot be maintained at or near 60 mm Hg despite inhalation of 100% O_2 or if there is progressive hypercapnia and a decline of arterial pH.

Morphine

- This agent continues to be an extremely valuable drug for the treatment of CPE. The drug not only diminishes the patient's distress but reduces the work of breathing. This is believed to be a result of the blunting of chemoreceptor-mediated ventilatory reflexes. Morphine achieves its hemodynamic effects by causing arteriolar and venous dilatation through its ability to diminish the vasoconstrictive effects of increased sympathetic tone. The precise site of vasodilatation produced by morphine is uncertain, but it is currently believed that morphine may act primarily by increasing the pooling of blood in the splanchnic circulation. Morphine sulfate is usually administered in doses of 3 to 5 mg intravenously over a 3-minute period. This dose may be repeated two or three times at 15-minute intervals. The patient should be monitored for respiratory depression, which can be reversed by the narcotic antagonist naloxone. Morphine should be avoided if the pulmonary edema is associated with hypotension, intracranial bleeding, disturbed consciousness, bronchial asthma, chronic pulmonary disease, or reduced ventilation—specifically in those patients with an increased arterial PCO_2.

Aminophylline

- Intravenous aminophylline is effective when bronchospasm and wheezing are present. Often, especially in the elderly, there may be a combination of bronchial asthma and CPE. Aminophylline is also a venodilator and has positive inotropic actions. The usual dose is 5 mg/kg administered over 15 minutes followed by an infusion of 0.5 to 0.9 mg/kg every hour. Care should be taken not to administer the drug too rapidly, because arrhythmias and hypotension can occur. Optimal blood levels range from 10 to 20 mg/L.

Treatment of Precipitating Factors

- In addition to applying the general measures discussed previously, attention should be accorded to identifying and treating the precipitating factors. Electrical cardioversion may be necessary, for example, when acute pulmonary edema is precipitated by a tachyarrhythmia and the increased heart rate is unresponsive to pharmacologic treatment. When CPE is precipitated or aggravated by a hypertensive crisis, the treatment is clearly directed at decreasing blood pressure by a rapidly acting hypotensive agent such as nitroprusside.

Preload Reduction

- A reduction of LV preload is highly desirable in patients with CPE, and it is primarily intended to shift central blood volume to the periphery, thus reducing end-diastolic volume and pressure.
- When acute HF is associated with an expanded circulating volume, as, for example, with acute exacerbation of chronic HF, substantial preload reduction can be achieved without a significant decline in arterial pressure.
- On the other hand, in the setting of acute HF and normovolemia (i.e., acute myocardial infarction), aggressive reduction in preload may lead to a significant decrease in cardiac output, especially in patients with normal or slightly reduced arterial pressures.

- It is, therefore, important to decide in advance whether the patient who presents with acute pulmonary edema is likely to be at increased risk of developing hypotension with reductions in LV preload. If there is uncertainty, pulmonary artery catheterization may be indicated in order to monitor and characterize hemodynamics and to guide therapy. LV preload can effectively be reduced by diuretics, venodilators, rotating tourniquets, or phlebotomy. The latter is seldom required today because of the effectiveness of the intravenously administered agents.

Diuretics

- Rapidly acting intravenous loop diuretics elicit a rapid diuresis in patients with pulmonary edema and reduce pulmonary venous pressure by reducing total blood volume. Loop diuretics may improve pulmonary congestion even before diuresis has occurred. These hemodynamic effects are the result of the direct peripheral arterial and venodilating actions of loop diuretics. It is now believed that vasodilatation, rather than diuresis, is the principal early mechanism by which symptoms are improved in pulmonary edema.
  - *Furosemide* is the most widely used loop diuretic in the treatment of CPE. The dose is determined by whether the patient has received prior diuretic therapy. In those patients who have had no prior exposure to diuretics, a dose of 40 to 60 mg administered intravenously over a 2-minute period will normally suffice, whereas patients who are treated chronically with diuretics and patients with impaired renal function may require doses of 120 to 200 mg intravenously.

Venodilators

Nitroglycerin

- This agent effects vasodilatation by stimulating guanylate cyclase within the vascular smooth muscle of arterial resistance and venous capacitance vessels. The predominant site of action depends on the amount of the dose being administered. At lower doses, nitroglycerin acts principally on the peripheral veins and, thus, reduces right and left ventricular filling pressures. At higher doses, nitroglycerin causes modest arterial vasodilatation; consequently, it may improve cardiac output. Additionally, nitroglycerin can reduce the degree of mitral regurgitation. Furthermore, nitrates reduce subendocardial ischemia by increasing coronary vasodilatation and by reducing myocardial oxygen requirements through unloading effects.

- Nitroglycerin is very effective in relieving the symptoms of acute pulmonary edema and is often the preload-reducing agent of choice for patients with underlying ischemic heart disease. Nitroglycerin should be administered in a manner that ensures the fastest onset of action. In general, the intravenous route is preferred. The initial infusion rate is commonly 10 μg/min, and the rate may be increased to 300 μg/min to achieve desired effects. As a general principle, the dose of nitroglycerin should not be increased when the systolic arterial pressure falls below 100 mm Hg. Tolerance has been demonstrated with all forms of nitroglycerin and is maximal after 16 to 18 hours of continuous administration. Sublingual administration (0.3 to 0.6 mg) of nitroglycerin also reduces LV preload, but buccal absorption may be erratic.

Recombinant Human BNP (Nesiritide)

- BNP increases glomerular filtration and inhibits sodium reabsorption, causing natriuresis and diuresis. This natriuretic peptide causes vascular smooth muscle relaxation with consequent arterial and venous dilation, leading to reduced blood pressure and ventricular preload. BNP also inhibits central and peripheral sympathetic activation and the renin-angiotensin-aldosterone axis.[1]
  - BNP infusion (nesiritide) has been shown to decrease pulmonary capillary wedge pressure and improved cardiac index and urinary flow rate in a dose-dependent manner.[2,3] Nesiritide lowers cardiac filling pressures without causing tachycardia or ventricular

arrhythmias. Favorable effects have been shown in the treatment of decompensated HF. The recommended dose of nesiritide is a 2 μg/kg intravenous bolus, followed by continuous infusion of 0.01 μg/kg/min, with optional titration to 0.03 μg g/kg/min. Uncertainties remain about the advantages of this drug over agents such as dobutamine and nitroglycerin. This agent may be best reserved for patients with acute HF who do not improve rapidly with standard therapy.

Afterload Reduction

- Ventricular afterload (systolic wall stress) has a major influence on ventricular systolic performance. As discussed earlier, ventricular afterload is increased in most patients with HF, and the detrimental effects of afterload excess are proportional to the degree of LV systolic dysfunction. Afterload reduction with vasodilator therapy is directed at reducing excessive LV wall stress with a resultant increase in stroke volume and a decrease in end-diastolic pressure. A reduction in afterload provides the greatest hemodynamic benefit for patients with the most advanced HF; a far greater increase in stroke volume and decrease in end-diastolic pressure is achieved with similar reductions in wall stress in patients with severe LV systolic dysfunction compared to patients with milder forms of HF.

Nitroprusside

- Intravenous nitroglycerin is usually the vasodilator of choice for most patients with HF and underlying ischemic heart disease, but nitroprusside is the vasodilator of choice when a substantial reduction in LV afterload is required. Although both vasodilators affect vascular smooth muscle, the actions of nitroprusside and nitroglycerin differ in important ways. Because the magnitude of arterial vasodilatation that is achieved with nitroprusside is greater than with nitroglycerin, nitroprusside has the greater potential to produce hypotension. Such hypotensive action may lead to more neurohormonal activation, and this may be the reason why rebound hemodynamic effects following abrupt withdrawal of the drug occur more frequently with nitroprusside than with nitroglycerin. Nevertheless, nitroprusside infusion improves ventricular performance by decreasing all the major components of LV afterload (systemic vascular resistance, arterial stiffness, arterial wave reflectance, and chamber size). In fact, proper dose selection achieves a reduction in afterload and preload with little change in systemic blood pressure.

- Nitroprusside is reserved for clinical situations requiring acute, short-term afterload reduction. The typical patient who may benefit from an infusion of nitroprusside has an elevated filling pressure (greater than 20 mm Hg), inadequate cardiac output with compromised peripheral perfusion, and a systemic arterial pressure that exceeds 90 mm Hg. This clinical scenario is frequently encountered among patients with a large myocardial infarction, decompensated chronic HF, or acute valvular regurgitation or, on occasion, following a cardiopulmonary bypass.

- It should be emphasized that nitroprusside represents a stabilizing pharmacological bridge to more definitive interventions (e.g., valve replacement or coronary revascularization). The end points of acute vasodilator therapy can vary somewhat from patient to patient, but reasonable hemodynamic end points include a reduction in LV filling pressure to approximately 15 mm Hg and an increase in cardiac output that ensures adequate tissue oxygen delivery (indicated by a cardiac index that exceeds 2.5 L/m^2/min) while maintaining a systemic blood pressure of approximately 90 mm Hg.

- The optimally effective and safe administration of nitroprusside often requires hemodynamic monitoring via intra-arterial and pulmonary artery balloon flotation catheters. The initial dose of 0.10 to 0.20 μg/kg/min is gradually increased as needed to attain the desired clinical and hemodynamic effects. Nitroprusside can effectively augment the hemodynamic effects of dopamine, dobutamine, and similar agents.

- The incidence of side effects and toxicity is directly related to the dose and duration of administration. Nitroprusside should not be withdrawn abruptly because of the danger of rebound hypertension. Cyanide may accumulate with prolonged high doses of nitroprusside and contribute to lactic acidosis. Toxicity can be avoided by monitoring blood lactate and thiocyanate levels.

Inotropic Support

- Positive inotropic agents are generally considered if the patient is not responding appropriately to vasodilators and there is significant systolic dysfunction or cardiogenic shock. Many positive inotropic agents, such as dobutamine and amrinone, not only improve LV systolic function but have a direct vasodilating effect on the peripheral vascular system. Under these circumstances, as mentioned earlier, invasive hemodynamic monitoring is usually indicated.

Dobutamine

- This beta-adrenergic agonist stimulates β_1-, β_2-, and α_1-adrenergic receptors. Cardiac contractility is increased by virtue of its β_1- and α_1-effects, but, because the α_1-adrenergic effects are generally counterbalanced by the β_2 actions, there is normally little change in blood pressure. Dobutamine markedly increases cardiac output but produces only modest changes in LV filling pressures. Heart rate generally only increases when doses greater than 10 μg/kg/min are used. Compared with dobutamine, dopamine is a better vasoconstrictor, and amrinone and milrinone are better vasodilators. Dobutamine can be combined with nitroglycerin, nitroprusside, dopamine, and amrinone to produce added hemodynamic benefits.
- The usual dose of dobutamine is 2.5 to 15 μg/kg/min. Short-term infusions are often extremely effective in the treatment of unstable acute HF, especially when systolic pressures are relatively preserved. Long-term infusion should be avoided because of the development of hemo-

dynamic tolerance. Dobutamine is likely to increase myocardial oxygen consumption and can potentially precipitate serious arrthyhmias.

Dopamine

- Physiologically, dopamine is the precursor of norepinephrine and releases norepinephrine from the stores of the nerve-endings in the heart. Dopamine has the valuable property in severe HF of specifically increasing renal blood flow by activating postjunctional dopaminergic receptors. This vasodilatory effect is observed at doses of 1 to 2 μg/kg/min and peaks at a dose of 7.5 μg/kg/min, and the vasoconstrictive effects begin at doses of 10 μg/kg/min or more.

- Because the inotropic effects of dopamine result primarily from its indirect effects, dopamine's use in advanced HF is limited by the neurotransmitter depletion present in the failing heart. In the milder forms of HF, dopamine may have effects similar to dobutamine, except for the greater tendency to increase heart rate and a tendency to increase systemic vascular resistance and ventricular filling pressures at medium and higher doses.

- Dopamine should be infused through a long indwelling line because of the risk of extravasation. Extravasation may cause necrosis and sloughing of the surrounding tissue (as a result of the vasoconstrictive effects of the agent). Infusion with dopamine should be started at doses no higher than 2 to 5 μg/kg/min and should not be increased beyond 5 μg/kg/min in patients with blood pressures of 100 mm Hg or higher. In markedly hypotensive patients with peripheral hypoperfusion, large doses of dopamine can be used to support systemic blood pressure, either alone or in combination with norepinephrine.

Amrinone and Milrinone

- These phosphodiesterase inhibitors produce dose-dependent increases in cardiac output and decreases in LV filling pressures as a result of the interaction of their positive inotropic, positive lusitropic, and peripheral vasodilator actions. The net result is a hemodynamic profile similar to the combination of nitroprusside and dobutamine. Because of their vasodilating effects, amrinone and milrinone are less likely than dobutamine to increase heart rate and myocardial oxygen consumption. Despite these theoretical advantages, myocardial ischemia has been provoked by these agents and marked hypotensive episodes have been observed.

- Therapy with amrinone is started as an initial bolus of 0.75 μg/kg, followed by an intravenous infusion of 5 to 20 μg/kg/min. Milrinone requires a loading dose of 50 μg/kg over 10 minutes, followed by a maintenance infusion of 0.375 to 0.75 μg/kg/min.

Choice of Therapeutic Regimen

- In choosing the appropriate regimen, it is helpful to classify patients into hemodynamic subsets. Much of the previous discussion emphasized the treatment of pulmonary edema in patients with predominant systolic dysfunction (i.e., pulmonary congestion with depressed systolic dysfunction). A second subset of patients with acute pulmonary edema is the group with normal or near-normal systolic dysfunction; such patients are generally said to have LV diastolic dysfunction. In others, systolic and diastolic dysfunction coexist. The initial treatment of congestive HF and pulmonary edema is similar, but some differences deserve mention.

Diastolic Dysfunction

- This hemodynamic subset consists of patients with elevated filling pressures (greater than 18 mm Hg) and preserved systolic function (normal or near-normal ejection fractions). The left ventricle is typically not enlarged, and cardiac output may be normal. Clinical evidence of pulmonary edema in a patient with echocardiographic evidence of hypertrophy and a normal ejection fraction can be taken as evidence supporting the diagnosis of diastolic dysfunction. Unless there is uncertainty regarding the hemodynamic subset, such patients usually do not require hemodynamic monitoring.

- A major goal of therapy is to reduce the left atrial and pulmonary venous pressures. Diuretics, venodilators, and other preload-reducing agents are used as discussed previously. The steep, stiff diastolic pressure–volume curve can be responsible for a substantial decrease in filling pressure with little change in volume; as a result, hypotension often occurs with the usual dose of diuretics. Thus, cautious administration of lower-than-usual doses of diuretics is advisable. Aggressive treatment of systemic, arterial hypertension often provides the prompt clearing of pulmonary edema. The conversion of an atrial arrhythmia to sinus rhythm can be equally beneficial. Finally, ischemia, if present, should be treated aggressively. The long-term therapy of diastolic dysfunction is beyond the scope of this chapter.

Systolic LV Dysfunction

■ This hemodynamic subset consists of patients with little or no cardiac enlargement, high filling pressures (greater than 18 mm Hg), depressed ejection fraction (less than 40%), and a low cardiac output (cardiac index of 2.2L/m^2/min or less). Among such patients, therapy is essentially the same as that for predominant systolic dysfunction. Those patients with a blood pressure of 90 mm Hg or higher are best treated initially with nitroprusside, dobutamine, or both. Dobutamine can significantly increase stroke volume and slightly decrease preload and afterload, and nitroprusside will further increase stroke volume and decrease the LV filling pressures. Alternatively, intravenous milrinone may be used to achieve similar hemodynamic end points. When the systolic blood pressure is lower than 90 mm Hg, the chance of survival is markedly decreased.

Treatment of the Underlying Condition

■ As stressed previously, the recognition of the underlying cardiac disorder is of utmost importance, because certain conditions may require semiurgent surgical correction (e.g., valve replacement for patients with acute mitral or aortic regurgitation).

■ Management Options in Chronic HF

Introduction

- Figure 5-1 outlines the various therapeutic options as they relate to the severity of HF.

Nonpharmacologic Management of HF

General Measures

- The successful management of the complex syndrome of HF depends not only on prescribing the appropriate medications but also on whether patients are able to comply with self-management strategies, such as the daily recording of body weight and other lifestyle changes. Such simple methods have been shown to decrease hospital readmissions and improve quality of life. Multidisciplinary HF programs have been developed to support these endeavors.[4,5] Several issues should be addressed.

Figure 5-1: Depicted is a schematic representation of the incremental use of pharmacologic, nonpharmacologic, and surgical modalities as they relate to the severity of HF. Patients with stage A HF are at high risk of HF but do not have structural heart disease or symptoms of HF. This group includes patients with hypertension (HT), diabetes (DM), coronary artery disease, hypercholesterolemia (hyperchol), previous exposure to cardiotoxic drugs, or a family history of cardiomyopathy. Patients with stage B HF have structural heart disease but have no symptoms of HF. This group includes patients with LV hypertrophy, previous myocardial infarction, LV systolic dysfunction, or valvular heart disease, all of whom would be considered to have New York Heart Association (NYHA) class I symptoms. Patients with stage C HF have known structural heart disease and current or previous symptoms of HF. Their symptoms may be classified as NYHA class I, II, III, or IV. Patients with stage D HF have refractory symptoms of HF at rest despite maximal medical therapy, are hospitalized, and require specialized interventions or hospice care. All such patients would be considered to have NYHA class IV symptoms. ACEI denotes angiotensin converting enzyme inhibitors; ARB, angiotensin receptor blocker; BiV, biventricular pacing; and VAD, ventricular assist device. Adapted from: Jessup M, Brozena S. Medical progress: heart failure. *N Engl J Med.* 2003;348:2007-2018.

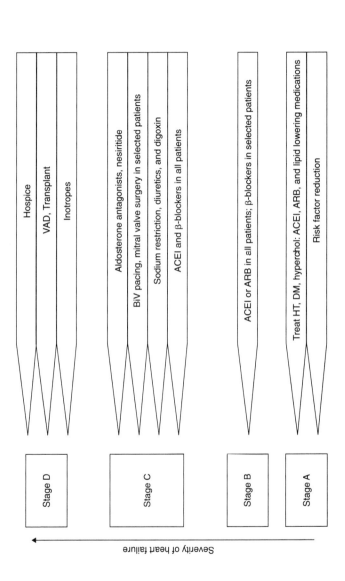

Severity of heart failure

Stage A
- Risk factor reduction
- Treat HT, DM, hyperchol: ACEI, ARB, and lipid lowering medications

Stage B
- ACEI or ARB in all patients; β-blockers in selected patients

Stage C
- ACEI and β-blockers in all patients
- Sodium restriction, diuretics, and digoxin
- BiV pacing, mitral valve surgery in selected patients
- Aldosterone antagonists, nesiritide

Stage D
- Inotropes
- VAD, Transplant
- Hospice

Compliance with the Treatment Plan

- Adherence to the treatment plan is crucial to the overall success of managing patients with HF. Factors that contribute to noncompliance include lack of knowledge, poor motivation, decreased understanding, lower perceived self-efficacy, forgetfulness, and insufficient support from family and other caregivers.
  - Compliance is achieved by educating the patient and family members about the progressive nature of HF and the symptoms and signs that indicate early decompensation, such as worsening dyspnea and an increase in weight of more than 3 lb over a 3-day period.

Dietary Restrictions

- Sodium intake should be restricted to no more than 2 g per day for patients with advanced HF. A 2-g sodium diet is unpalatable for some patients, whereas a 3-g sodium diet may be a more realistic target for patients with mild to moderate HF.
  - Patients should be advised to refrain from adding salt to food during preparation and to avoid canned and prepared foods. The use of salt substitutes and spices may be helpful.
- Water restriction is usually implemented for hyponatremic patients.
  - Limiting fluid intake to 2 L per day usually helps patients maintain weight and can reduce the need for large doses of diuretics in patients with advanced HF.
- Other dietary restrictions should be encouraged when there is evidence of lipid abnormalities in patients with ischemic cardiomyopathy and a reduced-calorie diet should be encouraged for obese patients. However, other patients with advanced HF can be anorexic and cachectic, which can be exacerbated by unnecessary dietary restrictions. Frequent, small meals may combat the effect of anorexia caused by congestion of the gastrointestinal tract.

Weight Reduction

- Markedly overweight patients may derive considerable hemodynamic and symptomatic benefit from weight reduction.

Avoidance of Alcohol and Tobacco

- Acutely, ethanol decreases myocardial contractility. The consumption of three or more drinks per day results in a dose-dependent increase in blood pressure, which returns to normal within weeks of abstinence. As a result, heavy drinking is an important contributor to mild to moderate hypertension. Chronic heavy drinking can cause cardiomyopathy, with symptoms ranging from unexplained arrhythmias in the presence of left ventricular impairment to heart failure with dilation of all four heart chambers and myocardial dysfunction. It is believed that up to one-third of cases of cardiomyopathy are alcohol-induced.
- One of the largest potentially modifiable risk factors to health, and especially to patients with HF, is the abuse of tobacco products.

Activities and Exercise

- Patients should be encouraged to stay as active as possible, including sexual activity and a moderate exercise regimen. The accumulated evidence to date suggests that aerobic exercise training by HF patients results in improved exercise duration, less fatigue, and improved general well-being. However, patients should be counseled to avoid lifting a significant weight (e.g., more than 20 lb) or performing exercises that cause strain.
- Sexual problems are well documented and should be carefully assessed. Fears about physical exertion or symptoms may contribute unnecessarily to sexual difficulties. Sexual practices may have to be modified to accommodate patients with limited exercise tolerance.

Referral to a Multidisciplinary HF Program

- Studies of other chronic illnesses, such as diabetes and asthma, support the notion that a chronic condition such

as HF is best managed by enrollment in a multidisciplinary HF program.[4,5] Many of these measures reduce
morbidity and are cost-effective.

Specific Nonpharmacologic Treatments for Systolic HF
Exercise Training

- Physical deconditioning plays a major role in the
  exercise- related symptoms of patients with HF. En-
  durance training can improve the functional work capacity of patients with chronic HF.[6] Training benefits have
  been attributed in particular to peripheral adaptations,
  including enhanced oxidative capacity of the working
  skeletal muscle and correction of endothelial dysfunction
  in the skeletal muscle vasculature.

- A review of the clinical evidence from existing trials suggests that exercise training of patients with HF seems to
  be safe and beneficial in improving overall exercise
  capacity, as measured by peak oxygen consumption, peak
  workload, exercise duration, and parameters of submaxi-
  mal exercise performance.

- For guidelines on the intensity and monitoring of exercise
  training, the reader is referred to the American Heart
  Association Committee on Exercise, Rehabilitation, and
  Prevention. Exercise and heart failure: a statement from
  the American Heart Association Committee on Exercise,
  Rehabilitation, and Prevention. *Circulation.* 2003;107:
  1210-1225.

Biventricular Pacing

- Left bundle branch block results in the loss of synchrony
  of ventricular contraction and impairs both regional and
  global LV systolic function. This loss of synchrony further impairs already poor systolic function in patients
  with ischemic and nonischemic cardiomyopathies. This
  electrocardiographic finding has been shown to be associated with adverse clinical outcomes. The prevalence of
  conduction delay in patients with HF is as high as 30%.
  Biventricular pacing has been shown to restore synchro-
  nous ventricular contraction and so improve overall LV
  systolic function. This technique involves the transve-
  nous placement of a third pacing lead via the right atrium

and coronary sinus into a LV cardiac vein; this is in addition to the standard pacing leads in the right atrium and right ventricle and permits simultaneous stimulation of the right and left ventricles.[7–9]

- Biventricular pacing appears to improve symptoms and decrease hospital admissions of HF patients with left bundle branch block, specifically those with moderate to severe chronic symptoms of HF (NYHA class III or IV) and a QRS duration of 130 ms or more.

- The response to biventricular pacing has been shown to be unpredictable and heterogeneous, and it raises the issue of how patients are selected.[9] Up to 30% of patients who receive a biventricular pacer do not improve. Electrocardiography has been shown to be a poor predictor of patients' responses. Other techniques, such as echocardiographic techniques using tissue Doppler imaging, may be used in the future to better select the patients most likely to respond.

- It seems reasonable to consider biventricular pacing as a form of therapy in symptomatic HF patients with an ejection fraction of 35% or less and a left bundle branch block with a QRS duration of 130 ms or more.

Sleep Apnea

- Sleep-related breathing disorders, including obstructive and central sleep apnea, often coexist with HF.[10] Epidemiologic studies suggest that the prevalence of obstructive sleep apnea varies from 11% to 37%. Moreover, having obstructive sleep apnea is associated with significantly increased odds of having HF. This obstructive sleep apnea can be relieved by therapy with continuous positive airway pressure, which leads to improved mortality and LV function.

Pharmacologic Treatment of HF

Stage A HF

- Treatment goals are as follows:

Modification of Risk Factors

- The aggressive treatment of risk factors (e.g., hypertension, coronary artery disease, and diabetes mellitus) has a favorable effect on reducing the incidence of adverse cardiovascular events in the future.

- It is recommended that the target for diastolic blood pressure in patients considered to be at high risk, particularly those with diabetes, be lower than 80 mm Hg. Treatment with ACE inhibitors has been associated with significant reductions in the rates of death, myocardial infarction, and stroke in asymptomatic patients at high-risk with diabetes or vascular disease and no history of HF. Angiotensin receptor blockade appears to delay the first hospitalization for HF of patients with diabetes mellitus and nephropathy.

Attenuation and Prevention of Adverse Chamber Remodeling

- The effective treatment of hypertension has been shown to decrease the occurrence of LV hypertrophy and cardiovascular mortality, as well as reduce the incidence of HF by 30% to 50%. In this regard, ACE inhibition or angiotensin receptor blockade should be given serious consideration in patients who are in stage A.

Pharmacology of ACE Inhibitors and Angiotensin Blockers

- *ACE inhibitors*: The angiotensin-converting enzyme is identical to kininase II, the enzyme responsible for the degradation of kinins. Thus, the primary actions of ACE inhibitors are to inhibit the production of angiotensin II and the degradation of kinins. As a result, ACE inhibition causes peripheral vasodilation not only by blocking the formation of angiotensin II but by enhancing kinin-mediated prostaglandin synthesis. The currently used ACE inhibitors, with their recommended target doses, dose adjustments, drug interactions, adverse effects, and contraindications, are shown in Table 5-1.

- Data further suggest that ACE inhibition may affect the course of HF by improving diastolic function, preventing progressive loss of myocardial cells, and attenuating adverse ventricular remodeling in response to pressure

Table 5-1:   ACE Inhibitors

Drug	Dose (mg)	Frq	Target dosage	Dose adjustments	Durg interactions	Adverse effects	Contraindications
ACE Inhibitor				■ Initiate with a low dose (e.g., 12.5 mg of captopril or 2.5 mg of enalapril) and then ↑ to target range within 1–4 wks. ■ Start at lower dose if Na$^+$ < 135 mmol/L. ■ Discontinue with progressive azotemia or intolerable cough.	■ Reduce diuretic dose if BUN and Cr ↑. ■ ACEI + K$^+$-sparing diuretics may ↑↑ K$^+$. ■ ASA or NSAID may counteract the beneficial effects of ACEI. ■ ACEI + vasodilators may cause hypotension.	■ Dizziness (3.3%) ■ Headache (5%) ■ Agranulocytosis* ■ ↑ BUN and Cr ■ Angioedema* ■ Nausea (1.4%) ■ ↑ K$^+$ (1%) ■ Cough (2–3.4%)	■ Prior ACEI anaphylaxis ■ Severe renal impairment ■ K$^+$ > 5.5 mmol/L
Captopril	6.25–150	3x/d	50 mg TID				
Enalapril	2.5–20	2x/d	10 mg BID				
Lisinopril	2.5–40	1x/d	—				
Ramipril	2.5–10	2x/d	5 mg BID				
Quinapril	5–20	1x/d	—				
Zofenopril†	—	—	30 mg BID				
Trandopril†	—	—	4 mg QD				

ACEI, angiotensin-converting enzyme inhibitor; ASA, aspirin; BID, twice a day; BUN, urea; Cr, creatine; d, day; Frq, frequency; NSAID, nonsteroidal anti-inflammatory drug; QD, four times per day; TID, three times per day; wks, weeks; *, rare complications; †, not approved by the FDA in the United States; ↓, decreased; ↑, increased.

overload or ischemic injury.[11] These actions of ACE inhibitors have translated into an improved survival in a broad spectrum of patients with myocardial infarction and HF, ranging from those who are asymptomatic with LV dysfunction to those who are symptomatic with advanced HF. In addition, ACE inhibitors improve the functional status of patients with HF, with 40–80% of patients showing improvement in NYHA functional class. It should be recognized, though, that improvement in exercise tolerance does not occur immediately after initiating therapy with an ACE inhibitor, despite early hemodynamic improvements. Rather, tolerance increases slowly, with the maximum benefit appearing after 3 to 6 months. All patients with HF should therefore be considered for such treatment even if they are asymptomatic. Of note is the fact that the clinical, hemodynamic, and prognostic benefits of ACE inhibitors may be attenuated by the coadministration of aspirin, which blocks kinin-mediated prostaglandin synthesis. It is not yet known whether aspirin should be discontinued or the dose should be reduced when given with an ACE inhibitor. All ACE inhibitors are similar in their therapeutic profile. However, when ACE inhibitor treatment is initiated in severe HF, the shorter-acting inhibitor, captopril, is preferred because it is less likely to be associated with prolonged hypotension and renal dysfunction than longer-acting agents.

- *Angiotensin receptor blockers*: The angiotensin receptor blockers that have been evaluated in large clinical trials are shown in Table 5-2, along with their recommended target doses, dose adjustments, drug interactions, adverse effects, and contraindications. Angiotensin II receptor blockers (ARBs) block the vasoconstrictor and aldosterone-secreting effects of angiotensin II by selectively blocking the binding of angiotensin II to the AT_1 receptor found in many tissues. ARBs do not inhibit ACE (kininase II, the enzyme that converts angiotensin I to angiotensin II and degrades bradykinin), nor do they bind to or block other hormone receptors or ion channels known to be important in cardiovascular regulation.

Table 5-2: Angiotensin Receptor Blockade

Drug	Dose (mg)	Frq	Target dosage	Dose adjustments	Drug interactions	Adverse effects	Contraindications
ARB:				■ Initiate with a low dose and then ↑ to target range within 1–4 wks. ■ Start at lower dose if Na^+ < 135 mmol/L.	■ Reduce diuretic dose if BUN and Cr ↑. ■ ARB + K^+-sparing diuretics may ↑↑ K^+. ■ NSAID may counteract the benefits of ARBs.	■ Dizziness ■ Headache ■ Agranulocytosis* ■ ↑BUN and Cr ■ Angioedema* ■ Nausea (1.4%)	■ Prior ARB anaphylaxis ■ Severe renal impairment ■ K^+ > 5.5 mmol/L ■ Pregnancy
Irbesartan	75–300	1x/d	75–150 mg				
Losartan	25–100	1x/d	50 mg QD				
Candesartan	4–32	1x/d	32 mg QD				
Valsartan	40–320	2x/d	80–160 mg BID				

ARB, angiotensin receptor blocker; BID, twice a day; BUN, urea; Cr, creatine; d, day; Frq, frequency; NSAID, nonsteroidal anti-inflammatory drug; QD, four times per day; wks, weeks; *, rare complications; ↓, decreased; ↑, increased.

Published guidelines indicate that these drugs should not be used as first-line therapy for HF of any stage but should be used only in patients who cannot tolerate ACE inhibitors because of severe cough. There is consensus that angiotensin receptor antagonists are a reasonable alternative to ACE inhibitors.

Stages B and C HF

- The goals of therapy for patients with HF and a low ejection fraction are to improve survival, slow the progression of disease, alleviate symptoms, and minimize risk factors. The cornerstones of the pharmacologic treatment of symptomatic HF are ACE inhibitors and β-blockers.
- ACE inhibitors should be prescribed to all asymptomatic and symptomatic patients (stage B, C, or D HF) who have an LV ejection fraction that is less than 40%.
- *Principles of ACE inhibitor therapy*[12]
  - The optimal dose of an ACE inhibitor is uncertain.
  - No difference in mortality has been shown between patients receiving high-dose ACE inhibitors and those receiving low-dose ACE inhibitors.
  - The initiated ACE inhibitor dose should be not up-titrated until a β-blocker is commenced in patients with stage C HF.
  - A rise in serum creatinine may occur after initiation of therapy in patients with congestive heart failure (CHF). This rise usually occurs promptly, is less than 10–20%, is not progressive, and is a consequence of the renal hemodynamic changes brought about by ACE inhibitor therapy. Risk factors that predict a decline in renal function are hyponatremia; high-dose diuretic therapy; diabetes mellitus; and the use of long-acting, converting enzyme inhibitors. Serum creatinine often stabilizes and may decline thereafter.
  - Although there is no serum creatinine level per se that contraindicates ACE inhibitor therapy, greater increases in serum creatinine occur more frequently when ACE inhibitors are used in patients with underlying chronic renal insufficiency.

- The occurrence of acute renal failure should prompt a search for systemic hypotension (mean arterial pressure less than 65 mm Hg), volume depletion, or nephrotoxin administration. An attempt should be made to correct or remove these factors. Consideration should also be given to high-grade bilateral renal artery stenosis or stenosis in a single kidney.

- ACE inhibitors should be discontinued temporarily while precipitating factors for acute renal failure are corrected; ARBs are not an appropriate substitute under these conditions. Once acute renal failure has resolved with correction of the precipitating factors, ACE inhibitor therapy can be reinstituted.

- Hyperkalemia is a potential complication of ACE inhibitor therapy, particularly in patients with diabetes or chronic renal failure. Monitoring of serum potassium early after the initiation of therapy, an appropriate reduction in dietary potassium intake, and avoidance of agents that can aggravate hyperkalemia (e.g., potassium-sparing diuretics, nonsteroidal inflammatory drugs, and cyclooxygenase-2 inhibitors) are recommended. The dose of the ACE inhibitor should be decreased when hyperkalemia is mild (K^+ = 5.5 to 5.9 mmol/L); with more severe hyperkalemia, kayexalate could be considered.

β-blockers

- The beneficial effects of β-adrenergic blockade include improvements in survival, morbidity, ejection fraction, remodeling, quality of life, the rate of hospitalization, and the incidence of sudden death. β-blockers are indicated for all symptomatic patients with HF in a stable condition.

- Relative contraindications include the following:
  - Reactive airway disease
  - Diabetes in association with frequent episodes of hypoglycemia
  - Bradyarrhythmias or heart block

- Carvedilol (a nonselective β-adrenergic blocker with α-blocking properties) and extended release metoprolol (β-1 selective blocker) are the only two β-blockers that are specifically approved for the treatment of HF in the United States.[13,14] A recent trial showed that carvedilol extended survival compared with short-acting metoprolol.[15] There have been no studies to date on the use of atenolol in patients with HF.

- *The principles of β-blocker therapy are as follows:*
  - All patients with HF and no contraindications to using β-blockers should receive β-blocker treatment in addition to standard therapy. β-blocker treatment should be initiated at low doses and titrated upwards slowly. The recommended starting dosage of carvedilol is 3.125 mg twice daily for 2 weeks. If this dosage is tolerated, it can then be increased to 6.25, 12.5, and 25 mg twice daily over successive intervals of at least 2 weeks. Maintain patients on lower doses if higher doses are not tolerated. A maximum dosage of 50 mg twice daily has been administered to patients weighing over 85 kg (187 lb) with mild to moderate HF. Although many patients may show transient worsening of symptoms and require increased diuretic therapy and/or a decrease in the dose of the ACE inhibitor during the first 2 to 4 weeks of treatment, symptomatic benefits usually appear after about 6 to 8 weeks.
  - If a patient with HF is hypertensive, carvedilol may be preferred over metoprolol, whereas when a patient has advanced lung disease, metoprolol may be the preferred agent. Metoprolol may be better tolerated in patients with borderline blood pressures.
  - Except for patients with borderline blood pressures, β-blockers, for the most part, can be initiated in the outpatient setting.
  - Educating the patient about the potential side effects that may be encountered during the initiation of a β-blocker is important to ensure that the patient will persist with the agent. Frequent office visits are often helpful in motivating patients to continue with this agent.

Digoxin

- This agent has now been shown to be relatively safe in patients with HF.[16] The addition of digoxin to ACE inhibitors and diuretics in patients with moderate and severe HF decreases the rates of worsening HF and hospitalization. This beneficial influence was mainly found in patients with advanced HF and dilated ventricles. Data suggest that the maintenance of a low serum digoxin concentration (less than 0.09 ng/ml) is as effective in reducing the rate of cardiovascular events as the maintenance of a higher concentration and is associated with a lower rate of toxic effects. Elderly patients and those with renal insufficiency are more prone to toxic effects.

- Digoxin therapy may be associated with an increased risk of death from many causes among women, but not men.
- Loading doses of digoxin are not generally needed. In the presence of normal renal function, the typical dose of 0.125 mg daily may be instituted.
- Usually after a week of treatment, a steady state is reached; the patient should be then questioned for symptoms of toxicity, and an electrocardiogram, a serum digoxin level, serum electrolytes, blood urea nitrogen (BUN), and creatinine should be obtained.
- There is a commonly observed and clinically important interaction between digoxin and amiodarone.

Diuretics

- These agents are extremely effective in the symptomatic treatment of HF when there is evidence of fluid retention. However, the use of non-potassium-sparing diuretics is associated with an increased risk of arrhythmic death in patients with systolic LV dysfunction. The deleterious effects of diuretics are likely to be mediated via electrolyte abnormalities and activation of the renin-angiotensin-aldosterone system.[17]

Characteristics of Diuretics

- Loop diuretics block the sodium–potassium–chloride transporter. The loop diuretics available for clinical use are furosemide, bumetanide, and torsemide (Table 5-3).[17]
  - The bioavailability of oral furosemide is about 50% (ranging from 10% to 100%), making it difficult to

Table 5-3: Diuretics

Class of diuretic	Oral dose range (mg)	Dose in HF (total daily dose—mg)	Side effects
Loop:			■ Alterations in glucose metabolism
Furosemide	20, 40, 50, 80	20–600	■ Blood dyscrasias
Bumetanide	0.5, 1, 2	0.5–10	■ Development of oliguria
Torsemide	5, 10, 20 100	200	■ Elevated BUN or creatinine
			■ Hyperuricemia
			■ Hypokalemia
			■ Hypomagnesemia
			■ Hypovolemia
			■ Ototoxicity
Thiazide:			■ Hyperglycemia
Chlorthalidone	15, 25	30–60	■ Hyperuricemia
Hydrochlorothiazide	50, 100	25–100	■ Electrolyte abnormalities
Chlorothiazide	25, 50, 100 250, 500	10–20 mg/kg/BID	■ Photosensitivity
Metolazone	0.5, 2.5, 5, 10	5–20	■ Vasculitis
			■ Muscle spasms
			■ Stevens-Johnson syndrome
Potassium-sparing:			■ Anorexia
Amiloride	5	5–20	■ Diarrhea
Triamterene	50, 100	200–300	■ Headache
			■ Hyperkalemia
			■ Nausea/vomiting

predict how much furosemide will be absorbed in an individual patient. Higher doses of furosemide may be required to be effective. The absorption of bumetanide and torsemide is nearly complete, ranging from 80% to 100%. Whereas the amount of loop diuretic absorbed is normal in patients with edema, absorption appears to be slower than normal in others, particularly those with decompensated HF. The plasma half-lives of bumetanide, furosemide, and torsemide are 1, 1.5, and 3–4 hours, respectively. The implication of a drug with a short half-life is that the pharmacologic effect dissipates before the next dose is given. During this time, the nephron avidly reabsorbs sodium, limiting the diuretic effect over a 24-hour period.

- Thiazide diuretics block the electroneutral sodium–chloride transporter. The most commonly used thiazide diuretics are chlorthalidone, chlorothiazide, hydrochlorothiazide, and metolazone (Table 5-3).
  - The bioavailability of thiazides varies from 30% to 75%. Thiazides are less effective in patients with renal insufficiency (creatinine clearance of less than 30 ml/min).
- The potassium-sparing diuretics amiloride and triamterene block apical sodium channels, whereas spironolactone blocks the aldosterone receptor at the distal nephron.

Diuretic Resistance

- There are two forms of diuretic tolerance: (1) Short-term tolerance occurs when the diuretic effect is attenuated after the first dose has been administered. This can be prevented by restoring the diuretic-induced loss of volume. (2) Long-term tolerance is observed after a prolonged administration of a loop diuretic leads to avid sodium reabsorption at more distal sites. This phenomenon argues for the use of sequential nephron blockade, using combinations of loop and thiazide diuretics in patients who do not have adequate responses to optimal doses of a loop diuretic.[17]

Principles of Diuretic Use

- Use diuretics in moderation; avoid excessive doses of any single drug.
- Thiazides are useful for the management of patients with mild fluid retention. Higher doses of thiazides are required for patients with renal insufficiency than for other patients.
- A loop diuretic is the diuretic of choice for patients with renal insufficiency and for patients with more than mild fluid retention.
- The diuretic response of loop diuretics is not necessarily increased by administering larger doses, but it may be increased by administering moderate doses more frequently.
- Make use of synergism by adding a thiazide when there is an apparent tolerance to loop diuretics. Use this diuretic regimen to achieve euvolia; once fluid retention is effectively treated, then sequential nephron blockade could be used as needed when a patient gains weight despite adequate doses of loop diuretics. Consider using hydrochlorothiazide combined with triamterene to prevent excessive potassium wasting. Metolazone, a potent thiazide, could be added to a loop diuretic when hydrochlorothiazide appears to be ineffective in promoting sodium excretion. This combination often causes severe electrolyte disturbances.
- For patients who have poor responses to intermittent doses of a loop diuretic, a continuous intravenous infusion can be tried.
- The role of the BNP analogue nesiritide in treating resistant fluid retention has not been established, but nesiritide holds promise when combined with loop diuretics.
- Monitor serum electrolytes; avoid uremia, hyponatremia, hypokalemia, and hypomagnesemia.
- Use diuretics in combination with an ACE inhibitor.
- The frequency with which electrolytes should be monitored during treatment with diuretics is dependent on the strength of the diuretics prescribed, the extent of

diuresis required, the pharmacologic actions of the agent chosen, and the underlying renal function. Biochemical studies once or twice per week will usually suffice for the majority of patients until the electrolytes are stable or the patient is on a stable dosage. Thereafter, electrolytes should be checked every time a higher dose of the existing diuretic is prescribed or a new agent is added.

Aldosterone Antagonists

- Aldosterone stimulates the retention of salt, myocardial hypertrophy, collagen synthesis and deposition, and potassium excretion. Spironolactone, an aldosterone antagonist, appears to exert mortality benefits to patients with advanced symptoms of HF—specifically, NYHA class III or IV symptoms.[18] Spironolactone may decrease collagen synthesis that promotes increased myocardial stiffness. Hyperkalemia is a potential serious side effect, especially in diabetics with renal failure. Painful gynecomastia occurs in 10–15% of men who take spironolactone. A new class of aldosterone antagonist, eplerenone, is currently being evaluated in patients with a recent myocardial infarction.

Other Vasodilators

- Apart from certain exceptions, directly acting vasodilator drugs are no longer regarded as first-line therapy for the long-term management of HF. These exceptions are cases of HF complicated by valvular insufficiency or intolerance to ACE inhibitors or angiotensin receptor blockers. Of the vasodilators, nitrates and hydralazine are the most commonly used in this setting. This practice is based on the data from the Veterans Administration Heart Failure I trial that showed that the combination of isosorbide and dinitrate-hydralazine improves survival and the symptoms of HF.[19] (Dosages are as follows: Isorbide dinitrate: up to 90 mg three times daily; Hydralazine: up to 75 mg four times daily.) Nitrates may be used as first-line therapy when HF is complicated by or attributed to myocardial ischemia. Hydralazine in combination with isosorbide dinitrate is usually well tolerated in the majority of patients with symptomatic HF and may be used as an alternative for patients with contraindications or intolerance to ACE inhibitors. It may be further useful for patients who remain symptomatic on ACE inhibitors, although no controlled trials with this combination of drugs have been performed. However, side effects may cause a significant proportion of patients to discontinue one or both of these medications.

Calcium Channel Blockers

- The negative inotropic effects of first-generation calcium antagonists have led to a strong recommendation against their use for HF. The second-generation calcium antagonists, however, such as felodipine and amlodipine, produce peripheral vasodilation without associated negative inotropic effects. These calcium blockers were recently evaluated in two controlled trials to assess whether they provide additional hemodynamic and survival benefits to patients already on ACE inhibitors. Amlodipine was shown to improve angina and HF symptoms without increasing mortality in patients with underlying ischemic heart disease.[20] Moreover, a survival benefit was shown in patients with nonischemic LV dysfunction. Felodipine likewise showed no adverse effects on survival in patients with ischemic heart disease and HF. These agents may therefore be useful for patients with HF and angina-like symptoms not controlled with nitrates or β-blockers.

Anticoagulant Therapy

- Based on the lack of data and on the findings of the two Veterans Administration Heart Failure trials that reported an embolic complication rate of below 2.5% per 100 patients years, the American Heart Association and the Agency for Health Care Policy and Research does not recommend routine anticoagulation for patients with HF unless there is history of recent pulmonary or systemic embolism, recent AF, or mobile LV thrombi.[21] It is further recommended that the international normalized ratio (INR) should be between 2 and 3. Older individuals with a decreased ejection fraction after a myocardial infarction deserve special mention, because these patients have a substantial risk of stroke up to 5 years after the acute event. Anticoagulant therapy may have a protective effect against stroke after myocardial infarction in this subset of patients.

Revascularization for HF

- Patients with ischemic cardiomyopathy and moderate to large segments of dysfunctional but viable (hibernating) myocardium have a high likelihood of improving LV function after revascularization.[22-24] Moreover, revascularization results in an improvement in symptoms with a better chance of long-term survival. Assessment of viability (hibernation) is used to guide therapy for patients with ischemic cardiomyopathy, and patients with viable myocardium should be considered for revascularization. It has also been demonstrated that patients with viable myocardium who are treated medically have an increased risk of future cardiac events compared to those treated with a revascularization strategy.[25]

- Surgical revascularization for patients with an LVEF of less than 20% to recruit hibernating myocardium is becoming commonplace. These patients are generally sicker and subject to more perioperative risk factors and, despite an increased hospital mortality of approximately 4% to 6%, they enjoy a 90% one-year survival rate and a 64% five-year survival rate.

- Percutaneous revascularization appears to be an acceptable alternative to surgery in selected patients with a markedly reduced ejection fraction.

Surgical Options for HF

- *Mitral valve repair*: Repair of the mitral valve in patients with primary and secondary severe mitral regurgitation and an LVEF of less than 30% has been shown to be safe (with an operative mortality of less than 5%) and results in symptomatic improvement.[25] The results appear to be more predictable in patients with a nonischemic cardiomyopathy than in those with an ischemic cardiomyopathy. Mitral annuloplasty is generally performed with a complete (encircling) ring that reduces the mitral annular ring and offers effective correction of mitral regurgitation.

- *Remodeling surgery*: Direct surgical restoration of LV geometry with a reduction in LV size and shape has evolved over the past few years from partial left ventriculectomy to a modification of the Dor procedure for LV aneurysm.[26,27] However, carefully controlled studies are lacking. A multicentered, randomized trial, sponsored by the National Institutes of Health, is planned for patients with HF and coronary artery disease amenable to surgical revascularization. For patients with reported LV dysfunction, surgical volume reduction and revascularization will be randomized to either surgical revascularization alone or surgical revascularization and surgical ventricular restoration to determine its impact on cardiac function and overall survival.

Stage D HF

Inotropic Agents

Bridge to Definitive Therapy or Recovery

- Inotropic support may be helpful for critically ill patients with clinical evidence of hypoperfusion.[28] Signs of hypoperfusion include obtundation, hypotension, oliguria, and abnormal liver enzymes. Inotropic therapy should be started without delay until the cause of shock is determined and definitive therapy is available. An example of this scenario may be when a patient with chronic HF becomes hypotensive in the setting of an acute myocardial infarction. This patient should be supported by inotropes and an intra-aortic balloon pump until a percutaneous intervention can be performed.
  - *Inotropic therapy directed at blood pressure support*: (See previous section on inotropic support.) Dopamine in medium to high doses, in which pressor

effects may dominate (5 to 25 μg/kg_/min), is useful in this setting. Dobutamine and especially milrinone are unlikely to improve blood pressure because of their vasodilating properties.

- *Inotropic therapy directed at cardiac output support*: Dobutamine is the first choice if inotropic support is necessary to improve cardiac output. Milrinone causes greater peripheral vasodilation. The choice between dobutamine and milrinone for a particular patient is largely based on whether drug-induced vasodilation is likely to be associated with hypotension. It has been suggested that patients receiving β-blockers may respond better to milrinone than to dobutamine when inotropic support is required. However, no comparative data are available to support this view.

Management of Decompensated Chronic HF

- *Scenario A: evidence of congestion and hypoperfusion*: Patients with marked fluid overload and evidence of hypoperfusion, such as a narrow pulse pressure and cold extremities, generally require inotropic therapy in addition to diuretics to restore compensation.

- *Scenario B: evidence of congestion without hypoperfusion*: There are no data to support the use of inotropic infusions for patients without evidence of hypoperfusion. The use of vasodilators in this setting may be more appropriate. Many patients presenting with relatively low cardiac outputs in this setting have markedly elevated systemic vascular resistance in addition to high intracardiac filling pressures. Nitroprusside and nitroglycerin may provide significant improvement in hemodynamics in this group of patients and in those with severe mitral regurgitation in whom these vasodilators, especially nitroprusside, markedly reduce the mitral regurgitant fraction. BNP (nesiritide) also appears to be effective in this setting. Randomized trials are needed before these practices are deemed to be standards of care.

- *Scenario C: congestion with impaired renal responses*: Some patients with adequate perfusion become less responsive to diuretic therapy. One contributing factor is low regional perfusion of the kidneys. When the initial diuretic response is inadequate despite continued increases in intravenous boluses or infusions of loop diuretics and the addition of thiazide diuretics, diuresis may frequently be enhanced by low-dose inotropic infusions. Although renal function improves in some patients during an infusion of nitroglycerin or nitroprusside, the improvement of renal function with vasodilators has been less predictable than with the inotropic agents. Nesiritide is associated with selective renal vasodilation and may be useful in this setting. A specific strategy for supporting renal function during diuresis has not been established.

Ventricular Assist Device

- The most important indication for a ventricular assist device (VAD) is a patient who is not expected to recover cardiac function and who requires mechanical support as a bridge to heart transplantation.[26,29] This surgical option gives patients the opportunity to wait at home for an acceptable donor, and avoids hypoperfusion of vital organs and major ventricular arrhythmia.
- Another VAD application is made for patients who require ventricular assistance to allow the heart to rest and recover its function; it serves as a bridge to myocardial recovery for patients with acute myocarditis or idiopathic dilatative cardiomyopathy.
- The practice of implanting a VAD as destination therapy has not been established.

Heart Transplantation

- In the absence of significant comorbid conditions, patients who are 65 years or younger with refractory HF symptoms and who receive optimal medical therapy by which reversible factors have been corrected (including ischemia) should be considered for heart transplant evaluation.[30] For critically ill patients who require prolonged hospitalization for inotropic support or VAD, eligibility is limited only by contraindications to transplantation (see Table 5-4). For patients who are less severely ill, greater

Table 5-4:   Exclusion Criteria for Heart Transplantation

- Age greater than 65 years
- Fixed pulmonary vascular resistance (greater than 6 Wood's units)
- Peptic ulcer disease or pulmonary infarct within 3 months
- Brittle diabetes or diabetes with end-organ damage
- Major debilitating comorbid disease
- Severe peripheral vascular disease or carotid disease
- Symptomatic hypertension on multidrug therapy
- Active infection
- Renal failure (creatinine level greater than 2.5 mg/dl or creatinine clearance less than 50 ml/min
- Severe liver dysfunction (bilirubin level greater than 2.5 mg/dl or transaminase level more than 2 times normal)
- Significant obstructive pulmonary disease (forced expiratory volume in 1 second less than 1 l/min)
- Intrinsic coagulation abnormalities
- HIV seroconversion
- Amyloidosis
- Excessive obesity (greater than 33% above ideal body weight)
- Evidence of tobacco or ethanol abuse
- History of severe mental illness or psychological instability

selectivity is needed, and a variety of guidelines have been proposed. The most common indications for transplantation are idiopathic dilated cardiomyopathy and ischemic heart disease with LV dysfunction, each of which accounts for nearly half of the transplant population in any given year. More information about heart transplantation can obtained from a publication of the American College of Cardiology and American Heart Association on the selection and prioritization of patients for this procedure.[31]

Management of Specific HF Syndromes

Diastolic HF

- The medical management of diastolic HF differs from that caused by LV systolic dysfunction. The approach to treatment is based on the following objectives:
  - Determine and treat the underlying cause (e.g., ischemia and hypertension)

- Restore sinus rhythm when appropriate
- Relieve venous congestion
- Promote relative bradycardia

■ The most effective treatment of diastolic HF is to address the underlying cause. In this regard, ischemia should always be suspected, especially among the elderly. No drug currently exists that has been shown to effectively improve isolated ventricular diastolic function. The American College of Cardiology/American Heart Association Task Force on Evaluation and Management of Heart Failure recommends only nitrates and diuretics for the treatment of symptomatic diastolic HF; neither agent affects diastolic function. When prescribing these agents, it should be understood that a small change in central blood volume can result in a substantial decrease in LV filling pressure among patients with stiff hearts. Aggressive diuresis or venodilatation may result in hypotension, and the cautious administration of lower-than-usual doses of diuretics is advisable. Other agents, such as β-blockers and calcium antagonists, may have theoretical appeal in the treatment of diastolic dysfunction, but there is little evidence that these agents improve symptoms or exercise capacity. Recent data suggest that patients with diastolic HF may derive benefit from angiotensin receptor blockade.[32]

■ Strategies to Reduce Hospital Readmissions and Length of Stay

■ Repeat hospitalizations of patients with HF are a relatively frequent occurrence within a short period of time following hospital discharge. In one recent study, the 3-month readmission rate was reported to be approximately 42%. Another study noted that slightly more than 40% of elderly Medicare beneficiaries were readmitted to the hospital at least once in the 6-month period following the index admission for HF. Approximately 17% of patients were readmitted two or more times to the hospital over this relatively short follow-up period. The medical costs of readmissions alone are likely to contribute to more than 50% of the total cost of treating HF. Another key determinant of hospital cost is the hospital length of stay.

- There may be several reasons for the high readmission rates. For example, in community hospitals in Canada during 1992 and 1993, only slightly more than half (53%) of patients hospitalized with HF received ACE inhibitors during their acute hospitalization. Moreover, these agents were used significantly less often in women and patients aged 70 and older. In addition, poor patient adherence to pharmacologic and dietary therapy is a common cause of readmission for HF.
- Several strategies have been employed to better manage HF, including the use of a multidisciplinary approach, the use of disease management programs, and the addition of a nurse practitioner to assist in managing patients. It is clear that programs that focus on patient education, self-monitoring strategies, and frequent contact with the patients by telephone are likely to be cost-effective by improving patients' outcomes with HF.

■ References

1.   de Lemos JA, McGuire DK, Drazner MH. B-type natriuretic peptide in cardiovascular disease. *Lancet*. 2003;362: 316-322.

2.   Silver MA, Horton DP, Ghali JK, Elkayam U. Effect of nesiritide versus dobutamine on short-term outcomes in the treatment of patients with acutely decompensated heart failure. *J Am Coll Cardiol*. 2002; 39:798-803.

3.   Publication Committee for the VMAC Investigators (Vasodilatation in the Management of Acute CHF). Intravenous nesiritide vs nitroglycerin for treatment of decompensated congestive heart failure: a randomized controlled trial. *JAMA*. 2002;287:1531-1540.

4.   Rich MW, Beckham V, Wittenberg C, et al. A multidisciplinary intervention to prevent the readmission of elderly patients with congestive heart failure. *N Engl J Med*. 1995;333:1190-1195.

5.   McAlister FA, Lawson FM, Teo KK, Armstrong PW. A systematic review of randomized trials of disease management programs in heart failure. *Am J Med*. 2001;110:378-384.

6. Belardinelli R, Georgiou D, Cianci G, Purcaro A. Randomized, controlled trial of long-term moderate exercise training in chronic heart failure: effects on functional capacity, quality of life, and clinical outcome. *Circulation.* 1999;99:1173-1182.

7. Saxon LA, De Marco T. Cardiac resynchronization: a cornerstone in the foundation of device therapy for heart failure. *J Am Coll Cardiol.* 2001;38:1971-1973.

8. Abraham WT, Fisher WG, Smith AL, et al. Cardiac resynchronization in chronic heart failure. *N Engl J Med.* 2002; 346:1845-1853.

9. Reuter S, Garrigue S, Barold SS, et al. Comparison of characteristics in responders versus nonresponders with biventricular pacing for drug-resistant congestive heart failure. *Am J Cardiol.* 2002;89:346-350.

10. Kaneko Y, Floras JS, Usui K, et al. Cardiovascular effects of continuous positive airway pressure in patients with heart failure and obstructive sleep apnea. *N Engl J Med.* 2003; 348(13):1233-1241.

11. Litwin SE, Katz SE, Weinberg EO, Lorell BH, Aurigemma GP, Douglas PS. Serial echocardiographic-Doppler assessment of left ventricular geometry and function in rats with pressure-overload hypertrophy: chronic angiotensin-converting enzyme inhibition attenuates the transition to heart failure. *Circulation.* 1995;91:2642-2654.

12. Schoolwerth AC, Sica DA, Ballermann BJ, et al. Renal considerations in angiotensin converting enzyme inhibitor therapy: a statement for healthcare professionals from the Council on the Kidney in Cardiovascular Disease and the Council for High Blood Pressure Research of the American Heart Association. *Circulation.* 2001;10:1985-1991

13. Packer M, Coats AJ, Fowler MB, et al. Effect of carvedilol on survival in severe chronic heart failure. *N Engl J Med.* 2001;344:651-658.

14. MERIT-HF Study Group. Effect of metoprolol CR/XL in chronic heart failure: Metoprolol CR/XL Randomised Intervention Trial in Congestive Heart Failure (MERIT-HF). *Lancet.* 1999;353:2001-2007.

15. Pooke-Wilson PA, Swedberg K, Cleland JG, et al. Comparison of carvedilol and metoprolol on clinical outcomes in patients with chronic heart failure in the Carvedilol or Metoprolol European Trial (COMET): a randomized controlled trial. *Lancet.* 2003;362:7-13.

16.   The Digitalis Investigation Group. The effect of digoxin on mortality and morbidity in patients with heart failure. *N Engl J Med.* 1997;336:525-533.

17.   Brater DC. Diuretic therapy. *N Engl J Med.* 1998;339: 387-395.

18.   Pitt B, Zannad F, Remme WJ, et al. The effect of spironolactone on morbidity and mortality in patients with severe heart failure. *N Engl J Med.* 1999;341:709-717.

19.   Cohn JN, Johnson GR, Shabetai R, et al. Ejection fraction, peak exercise oxygen consumption, cardiothoracic ratio, ventricular arrhythmias, and plasma norepinephrine as determinants of prognosis in heart failure: the V-HeFT VA Cooperative Studies Group. *Circulation.* 1993;87(suppl): VI5-V16.

20.   Packer M, O'Connor CM, Ghali JK, et al. Effect of amlodipine on morbidity and mortality in severe chronic heart failure: Prospective Randomized Amlodipine Survival Evaluation Study Group. *N Engl J Med.* 1996;335: 1107-1114.

21.   Konstam M, Dracup K, Baker D, et al. *Heart Failure: Evaluation and Care of Patients with Left Ventricular Systolic Dysfunction.* Rockville, MD: Agency for Health Care Policy and Research and the National Heart, Lung, and Blood Institute, Public Health Service, US Department of Health and Human Services; June 1994. Clinical Practice Guideline, No. 11 (amended) AHCPR publication 94-0612.

22.   Kron IL, Flanagan TL, Blackbourne LH, Schroeder RA, Nolan SP. Coronary revascularization rather than cardiac transplantation for chronic ischemic cardiomyopathy. *Ann Thorac Surg.* 1989;210:348-352.

23.   Dreyfus G, Duboc D, Blasco A, et al. Coronary surgery can be an alternative to heart transplantation in selected patients with end-stage ischemic heart disease. *Eur J Cardiothorac Surg.* 1993;7:482-487.

24.   Luciani GB, Faggian G, Razzolini R, Livi U, Bortolotti U, Mazzucco A. Severe ischemic left ventricular failure: coronary operation or heart transplantation? *Ann Thorac Surg.* 1993;55:719-723.

25.   Allman KC, Shaw LJ, Hachamovitch R, Udelson JE. Myocardial viability testing and impact of revascularization on prognosis in patients with coronary artery disease and left ventricular dysfunction: a meta-analysis. *J Am Coll Cardiol.* 2002;39:1151-1158.

26. Vitali E, Colombo T, Fratto P, Russo C, Bruschi G, Frigerio M. Surgical therapy in advanced heart failure. *Am J Cardiol.* 2003;91:88F-94F.

27. Starling RC, McCarthy PM, Buda T, et al. Results of partial left ventriculectomy for dilated cardiomyopathy: hemodynamic, clinical, and echocardiographic observations. *J Am Coll Cardiol.* 2000;36:2098-2103.

28. Stevenson LW. Clinical use of inotropic therapy for heart failure: looking backward or forward? Part I: inotropic infusions during hospitalization. *Circulation.* 2003;108:367-372.

29. Zeltsman D, Acker MA. Surgical management of heart failure: an overview. *Annu Rev Med.* 2002;53:383-391.

30. Mudge GH, Goldstein S, Addonizio LJ, et al. 24th Bethesda conference: cardiac transplantation. Task Force 3: recipient guidelines/prioritization. *J Am Coll Cardiol.* 1993;22:21-31.

31. Costanzo MR, Augustine S, Bourge, et al. Selection and treatment of candidates for heart transplantation: a statement for health professionals from the Committee on Heart Failure and Cardiac Transplantation of the Council on Clinical Cardiology, American Heart Association. *Circulation.* 1995;92:3593-3612.

32. Yusuf S, Pfeffer MA, Swedberg K, et al. Effects of candesartan in patients with chronic heart failure and preserved left-ventricular ejection fraction: the CHARM-Preserved Trial. *Lancet.* 2003;362:777-781.

Index

Note: Page numbers with *f* indicate figures, *t* indicate tables.